This page ı

DROP

THE

S

DROP
THE
S

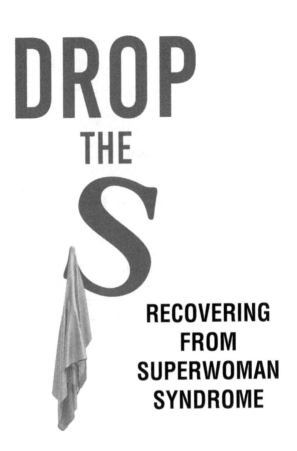

RECOVERING
FROM
SUPERWOMAN
SYNDROME

DR. MARYBETH CRANE

STONEBROOK
PUBLISHING

Stonebrook Publishing
Saint Louis, Missouri

DEDICATION

For my daughters, Alexandra, Caitlin, and Sasha.
I love you each unconditionally.

You are the best thing I've ever done with my life.

CONTENTS

AUTHOR'S NOTE

The purpose of this book is to provide a roadmap to healing for professional women who feel trapped in their own success, allowing them to ditch the Superwoman Syndrome and find physical, mental, spiritual, and financial wellness.

THE EVOLUTION OF SUPERWOMAN SYNDROME

A glance back over the last two decades was like an old movie with lots of static and distorted frames about what had to be somebody else's life. The old projector rattled away as it struggled with the dried-out tape. The movie skipped, and the picture came in and out of focus. There were so many jumbled pieces that it was difficult to make out the image. I needed a pause button or a hypothetical rewind. I needed to breathe and see if I could revamp the woman I'd become before I destroyed myself.

> *I had it all. Or at least I thought I did. I was Superwoman.*

I had it all. Or at least I thought I did. I was Superwoman. Even as a young girl, my parents taught me that I could do anything, and I could have it all. I believed it! My generation of women broke the glass ceiling in every profession. Progress in gender equality was extensive.

When I was a young girl, I envisioned the perfect happy life. Rural Rhode Island in the 1970s and 1980s was full of century-old homes with peeling paint and weathered, hardworking people who lived paycheck to paycheck. Despair was in the air, especially when the local shipyard was on strike—again. I worked very hard to get out of that lower-middle-class neighborhood full of discouraged people who didn't believe in their dreams anymore and stifled mine.

I always wanted to be a doctor. I was fascinated by being able to fix things, especially people. I thought doctors never had to worry about money and that everyone loved them. They never went on strike and could always find work, an important thought in the early '80s. I was taught that you would be happy if you have a purpose, enough money, and friends.

Money was the center of the daily arguments in our house. As a small child, I heard my parents argue about how my father spent too much money on things my mother thought were unnecessary. She was worried about paying the mortgage and making sure we had enough to eat. There was always enough, but she worried that something would happen, and we wouldn't be able to stay in our home, the only house we ever owned. Since money was scarce, I knew I had to earn a scholarship to college and get the hell out of that town. So, I did.

By thirty-five, I had everything I thought I wanted. A loving husband, a beautiful growing family, a lovely home, and a great professional career. Why wasn't I happy? I'd reached the Superwoman status of my dreams. The only problem was that the perfect life I'd envisioned wasn't sustainable, and I felt like I was drowning instead of swimming with the current. I was exhausted.

It wasn't one thing that brought me to my knees; it was the cumulative effect of my crushing responsibilities—the snowball that turned into an avalanche. I fell apart slowly, piece by piece, over several years until I no longer recognized myself.

I knew I wasn't the only middle-aged woman to feel this way. Superwoman Syndrome was and is an epidemic in our generation. So much for gender equality. We were expected to do it all!

I've always been a type-A personality, career-driven, and insanely competitive. I knew I could have it all, and I drove myself hard to be the best at everything. I built a multi-million-dollar podiatry practice from nothing—with my mom answering the phones—ran multiple marathons, finished two full Iron Man triathlons, and had three daughters to raise at the same time.

> *It wasn't one thing that brought me to my knees; it was the cumulative effect of my crushing responsibilities—the snowball that turned into an avalanche.*

In 2003, I even found the perfect business partner in the insanely driven Lori Cerami. Lori was my office administrator, and as we developed our relationship for over fifteen years, she came to know me better than I knew myself. We were a formidable power couple when our A-game was going strong. We weren't only business collaborators, but best friends.

With my two daughters, Alex and Caitlin, and Lori's daughter, Elise, in playpens, we worked side by side to build my company. From day one, Lori said she wouldn't work *for* me but would work *with* me. I treated her as an equal, and we shared our success. Lori was a fantastic business teammate and we worked forty- to sixty-hour weeks for more than fifteen years. Other doctors came and went, but Lori and I always ran the show. We had no idea that our driven personalities would eventually cause our burnout. Lori and I believed we could do anything and everything together.

But life sometimes throws you curveballs. We'd been having some financial trouble at home because my husband's business wasn't doing well. So in 2005, I took on extra lecturing because it was very lucrative. I was pregnant at the time, but I promised my doctor I'd stop traveling at twenty-five weeks. I didn't make it that far.

At twenty-four weeks, I was lecturing in Nashville when the baby stopped moving. I was so tired that I didn't notice until the next morning when my ankles swelled up, and I didn't feel well. I hopped on a plane to go home and went straight from the airport to my doctor, but it was too late. There was no heartbeat.

I was inconsolable. The baby was so big that I had to deliver him, and I thought I would die from the grief. My chest hurt, and I felt like I couldn't breathe. Riddled with guilt, I felt like I'd killed my son.

But life sometimes throws you curveballs.

Two weeks later, my oldest daughter asked her dad, "When is Mommy going to stop crying?"

The next day, I got up, put on my big girl pants, and went back to work.

Work was always my oasis. It was the place where I was in charge and had control, or at least the illusion of control. At work, I was Dr. Crane; at home, I was Mommy or Marybeth, and I felt like a slave to the life I'd created. I never felt like I had any control over my personal life. I felt like a failure because my kids weren't perfectly behaved or super-smart, and I had lost my son.

My daughters would say that, in those days, I was a raging lunatic when they misbehaved. My parents had taught me that children should be seen and not heard—a notion that didn't work in my household. I wanted my kids to feel loved and supported. No pressure to be perfect, but I wanted them to be perfect anyway.

In 2006, I gave birth to another daughter, Sasha, the baby I so desperately wanted after losing her brother. She was a very fussy baby. She was also a very tiny four-and-a-half pounds. I spent four months at home with her before going back to my practice. My partners covered for me because they knew how devastated I was when I lost my son, but I needed a paycheck after four months. So, I left Sasha with my mother; my precious, tiny baby was too small for daycare. Staying home was never a financial option. Although, for the first time in my life, I wanted to stay home and be a mom. So, I went back to work to make money to maintain our lifestyle. I felt trapped and angry.

And my husband's failing business wasn't improving. Jim ran a soccer center that also had a bar. That meant that he'd close the bar at 2:00 a.m., and he sometimes wandered home around 6:00 a.m. when I was getting up. I had no idea what he did between closing and 6:00 a.m. I didn't even ask. Then he'd sleep all day until he opened up the soccer center in the afternoon. That's when my resentment started to build.

Over the next three years, we drifted further and further apart. I don't think Jim ever understood that I was becoming more and more distant because I felt more and more helpless. He wasn't a lot of help around the house or with the girls. He was fun Dad; I was homework Mom. We no longer saw much of each other, and I didn't care. I felt empty and abandoned.

We weren't intimate except on a rare occasion when one of us needed it, and I'd started traveling again to lecture in other cities. I was so desolate and lonely that one evening after a conference, I fell into a colleague's arms. We were in similar situations at home, and we bonded over that pain. My infidelity and lies led to more guilt. I was anxious all the time. My chest ached with regret. Of course, Jim found out because I was too transparent and didn't lie well. He had a retaliatory affair and continued staying late at the soccer center almost every night. After a while, I realized my tumultuous marriage was the source of my crippling anxiety.

I went to see Dr. Peters, a marriage and family therapist. She was very helpful in helping me understand the family dynamics that led to our infidelity and collective misery.

She said, "Jim is like an employee of the marriage where you're the owner. He does just enough so you won't fire him. You, on the other hand, are fighting for the perfect family unit you've created in your head. You're so goal-oriented, you won't give up—even when you're drowning."

"I see what you mean," I replied. "I've put up with a lot. If I'm honest, I haven't felt like I had a partner since our second daughter was born."

"How do you feel about that? Why have you given Jim so much of your power in the relationship?" Dr. Peters inquired.

"I feel alone, anxious, and angry. I'm ready for a change, but I'm scared. I can't live like this. I need to take my power back. I support everyone financially and emotionally, yet feel no support from my partner. It's not about who makes more money. It's that I make all the money *and* feel like I do everything else for the family. Why am I married?"

"That, my dear, is a question only you can answer. I can help you either way," she said with a deep sigh.

Our marital angst and arguments continued, and the stress was palpable. I knew the right answer for me. It was time for us to part ways. But I didn't want to admit another failure.

We divorced in 2009 when Sasha was three years old. Alex was twelve, and Caitlin was ten. Neither of them understood why Daddy moved out and went to live with his parents, who lived only about a mile from our home. They cried a lot, and I tried to be everything for everyone. Jim wasn't helpful in the practical sense and didn't even try to help with the girls' expenses. Some things didn't change. He didn't have any money, so it was up to me to keep the family fiscally viable and the girls' lives as normal as possible. I was still trapped.

Just when I thought I was a master juggler, all the balls I had in the air started to drop. Alex never forgave me for throwing out her father. She thought I was the bad person, and her dad didn't do anything to discourage her from feeling that way. It was a tumultuous time for us. We had many discussions and arguments—what to eat for dinner, where to go on vacation, and whether the sky was blue—no matter what we talked about, Alex and I could never agree. She was confrontational about everything, screaming that I didn't understand or that I was stupid. There was one instance when I became a person I didn't even recognize. She'd called me a fucking bitch, and I'd had enough. I slapped her. There's no excuse for my behavior, but I was at my wit's end. Alex hated me. I felt like another chunk of me had died, that I'd lost

> *Just when I thought I was a master juggler, all the balls I had in the air started to drop.*

7

another child. Dr. Peters told me Alex would come to understand when she was older, but at the time, I didn't believe it.

Divorce is hard for anybody, but it took a heavy toll on me because I felt like I'd failed to hold it together. I was seething with anger toward Jim for his behavior during the breakup, which drove me to work more and more. I felt like if I built the practice and made more money, it would help repair the damage. If I supported the girls in the manner they were accustomed—or even better—they'd be all right in the long run. Work was something I was good at, and it gave me a sense of control.

Life did seem to calm down for a few years. Alex was safe, although I didn't have much of a relationship with her. Slowly, she was becoming less adversarial but certainly not warm. Caitlin and Sasha were the center of my life, and my practice was thriving.

Then the unthinkable happened. Lori's daughter, Elise, drowned at swim practice. She had been very close with my daughter, Caitlin, and she spent a lot of time with my family since Lori and I worked so much. Elise was thirteen years old when she died. I was there the day Elise was born, and I was in the ICU the day she died. That day, I not only lost another child but I felt like I lost Lori as well.

Lori and I were both in a fog of grief. I did what I needed to do. I propped up Lori and her family and helped plan a funeral and public memorial. I went to work organizing, something I was very good at, and it distracted me from the terrible truth of what had happened. It helped me dissociate from the grief for a time.

Lori's grief was overwhelming and persistent. She was a shell of her former self. But I couldn't let both of us fall apart; we had a business to run. I internalized my grief and went to work fixing everything for everybody. For the next two years, I did my job and either delegated Lori's responsibilities or picked up the slack for what she wasn't yet able to do. Then the exhaustion set in.

You can't fix grief; it's pernicious. It eats at your soul, and seemingly innocuous events trigger the sadness. I was thoroughly exhausted, drained of all energy, and without joy. What had happened to that vibrant, amazingly competitive woman who strove to be the best at everything? I used to feel ten feet tall and bulletproof. I could do everything for everybody and remain standing with a smile on my face. I used to set the world on fire and leap tall buildings in a single bound. I was the proverbial Superwoman!

> *You can't fix grief; it's pernicious. It eats at your soul, and seemingly innocuous events trigger the sadness.*

In late 2017, I went to my doctor and declared that there was something wrong with me. That's when I realized that I needed to drop the "S" from my chest.

2

I'M SO TIRED

'd always prided myself on being able to multitask. But that was only another lie I told myself. What I thought was multitasking was actually a lightning-speed juggling act that I kept up for years . . . until I couldn't. Just when my teenagers were at the height of their hormonal behavior, and I was in my mid-forties, I felt ready to collapse. I was so tired, but I didn't know why. It was a bone-weary, "I've been run over by a truck" exhausted feeling that never left me, even after a good night's sleep.

Before I realized I had a problem, my typical day looked something like this: I jolted awake at 5:30 a.m. My head was fuzzy, but I jumped out of bed anyway. I threw exercise clothes on and was out the door. My thirty-minute run felt like a chore. My legs were tired, but the run seemed to clear my head a bit. Back to the house by 6:00 a.m. to make lunches for my tribe before they woke up. I grabbed a cup of coffee and scarfed down a little breakfast while making breakfast for the kids and kissing my new husband goodbye. The dishes in the sink and piles of laundry would have to wait. It was time to get the kids up.

Whining and crabby, they finally made their way downstairs to eat breakfast, and I could hop in the shower, confident they were upright. I got ready for work while yelling for them to get their stuff together and brush their hair and teeth. Then it was time to walk out the door.

Three out of five days a week, they missed the bus, so I fought the traffic and dropped them off at two or three different schools, then sped to work and slid in the back door about ten minutes *after* my first patient was scheduled.

The office was the usual madness. Some days were organized chaos. Other days, I felt like I was running a kindergarten. Every once in a while, it was a well-oiled machine. I worked at my desk or had a meeting through my lunch hour, then saw more patients. I tried to get all my charts done before leaving, but that usually didn't happen. So, I rushed out the back door with barely enough time to meet my kids at the bus stop or pick them up at school if they'd missed the bus or had an afterschool activity. Then it was homework—why did I feel like I was taking algebra for the fourth time?—and more yelling.

Then I slapped something together for dinner, and finally, I sat down to watch a mindless ballgame or read a book. Of course, I had a cocktail or two or five. That was if the kids didn't have an extra activity or forget a project that was due the next day—or I didn't have a conference call. I got the kids bathed and ready for the next day, then off to bed they went.

I refilled my wine glass and wondered why I was so exhausted.

On the weekends, I was the social chairman, chief dishwasher, meal prepper for the week, laundry fairy, bookkeeper, travel agent, event planner, grocery shopper, and head referee.

So, why was I tired? Because it was impossible to keep up the Superwoman persona over an extended period of time.

But that didn't mean I slowed down. I was still navigating my daily life, seeing patients, running the practice with Lori back at my side, being Mom, and taking care of everyone around me. My check engine light was on, and I was ignoring it. I thought the problem might be the combination of early menopause and being overwhelmed by all my responsibilities, not to mention the never-ending roller coaster of grief, stress, and change. The last fifteen years had tested my resolve and my ability to do it all.

> *My check engine light was on, and I was ignoring it.*

"Crane," Lori yelled over to me, "What the hell's wrong with you? You've been a cranky bitch all week, and I'm over it! I had to talk Anna off the ledge because she wanted to quit after you yelled at her yesterday."

"I'm not that bad. She's too sensitive to criticism," I replied, then yawned for what must have been the hundredth time that morning. "I just need another cup of coffee and a competent assistant."

"I don't think coffee's going to fix this," Lori said. "You've been irritable and dragging ass for months. This week you've been particularly snarky. If you don't get your head out of your ass, more employees will flee the building. I can't keep up with the HR as it is."

"I'll try to get some more sleep this weekend. I'm just so busy with patients, charts, and keeping up with the kids. I'm exhausted," I replied with a heavy sigh.

"Seriously, Crane, I think there's something more going on with you. Have you seen the doctor lately?" Lori inquired.

"No. I don't have time for that. I'm fine," I answered as I gazed at the avalanche of papers on my messy desk.

"You're not fine, and you know it. I'll be the next one to quit if you can't figure it out. I don't think I even like you anymore," Lori said as she walked out of our joint office and slammed the door.

"Wow!" I said to the closed door.

I knew something was wrong but chose to ignore the warning signs. I would sleep ten or twelve hours on the weekend but wake up just as tired as the day before. My head was cloudy, my hair had thinned, I had no sex drive, and I woke up several times a night. I couldn't fall asleep without a glass or two of wine—or maybe the whole bottle. It was a never-ending cycle of caffeine in the morning, perhaps a little more in the afternoon, then wine after dinner to reverse the process in order to go to sleep. On top of all that, I didn't feel like doing *anything*. Including running! After forty years of competitive distance running, more than thirty marathons, and two full Ironman Triathlons, something was seriously wrong when I didn't want to run. Heck, I didn't want to exercise at all. Too tired for that. I also noticed a subtle change in my body. I was gaining weight in places I never had before. An extra ten pounds had crept onto my tiny frame.

Everything was spiraling downward, yet I was still trying to keep up the Superwoman persona.

Everything was spiraling downward, yet I was still trying to keep up the Superwoman persona. I pushed through the fatigue and other pain. I was an Ironman triathlete after all, which proved I could do almost anything, right? So, I donned my mask of perfection and kept on trucking.

Then I started noticing other symptoms. I had significant problems thinking, and I experienced an overall malaise. I was becoming forgetful. It wasn't the first time Lori pointed out that I was very confrontational and a total bitch to pretty much everyone. I'd get home from work exhausted, cook dinner, help with homework, and get the kids situated, but it wasn't pretty. Screaming at my kids to get their stuff done had become the norm.

My plate was full, and I didn't have time to feel bad or be sick or whatever this was. After everything I'd been through in the last few years, could it be that I was now depressed?

When Lori came back in with more stacks of paperwork, I was ready to talk.

"I think you might be right," I said. "I know something's wrong, but I don't have the time to make appointments and address it."

"If you don't try to figure out what's wrong, it may be too late," Lori answered. "And I'm serious about quitting if you continue to snap at me. I don't want to look for another job. No one else understands what I've been through. What we've been through. We've spent too much time and energy building this place together to let it fall apart.

"Let's get you fixed. Or at least figure out what's wrong. I'm calling that therapist you saw after the divorce. I think it was Dr. Peters, right? Maybe you're depressed?"

"I'm not depressed!" I yelled. "I'm just tired, and yes, I'm sorry I've been such a bitch lately. I'll go talk to Anna and see if I can repair that relationship."

14

"Forget about Anna. She'll get over it because she loves working with you when you're your normal self," Lori replied. "If you don't think you're depressed, maybe you should call your doctor and get a physical."

"Okay. I'll put it on my to-do list," I conceded.

"Put it at the top!" she retorted.

Whoa! What was that? I thought, feeling a little lightheaded, my heart racing.

I steadied myself on the counter in the empty exam room. It was near the end of a busy day, and I was tired. Feeling a little nauseous, I sat down in the exam chair.

I just need a minute to catch my breath, I told myself. *No reason for alarm.* My heart fluttered again, then skipped a beat or two. Was I having a heart attack? Was this how my life was going to end? In my office? I was too young for this!

Another wave of nausea crashed over me. I put my head between my legs. My heartbeat seemed to slow down, and I felt better. I sat up, and the spots in front of my eyes cleared. I slowly walked out of the exam room into the hall. The office was bustling; no one noticed my brief absence.

Time to act like everything was normal. I took a deep breath and continued like nothing had happened.

Deep down, I knew my problem, whatever it was, was getting serious. This was the third time this month that I'd almost passed out, and this time it was worse. I had to stop ignoring the signals. Time to make an appointment to investigate my fatigue and other symptoms. The therapist could wait. There was obviously something physically wrong with me.

15

I visited my friend, Dr. Reed, who'd been my OB/GYN and friend for the last twenty years or so. She was the same doctor who cried with me when my son was stillborn and rejoiced with me when Sasha was born. I described my symptoms and the dizzy episodes.

"Either I'm crazy, going through early menopause, or there's something really wrong with me," I said.

I was ready to hear that I had leukemia or Lou Gehrig's disease. Anything to explain why I was so exhausted all the time.

We discussed all the possible differential diagnoses for profound fatigue. We talked through a troubleshooting workup to find a medical reason. We also discussed psychological and hormonal factors that caused fatigue. Finally, because she'd been my friend for years and had known the roller coaster of my past few years, she suggested that I might be suffering from stress overload, burnout, and adrenal fatigue.

"Marybeth," she said as she sat back in her chair and took a long, deep breath, "You and I had this discussion right after you lost your son. Do you remember? I know it was a stressful time, so maybe it isn't ringing any bells."

"The months surrounding his death are a blur," I replied. "Can you refresh my memory?"

"We talked about physician burnout and adrenal fatigue. At the time, I was concerned that you were already in the first or second stage of burnout. You know, the honeymoon phase, when you think you can do it all? In women, we call it Superwoman Syndrome. That's when you're on an 'I can do everything' high. It's usually followed by the 'balancing act,' in which you start to unravel while you're on the high bar trying to do it all," she continued.

I started to play with my hair and fidget. This was getting uncomfortable.

"Yes, I remember you mentioning it, but I didn't take you seriously. I thought I was tired from all the mental trauma. Burnout is for mental midgets," I answered.

"No, it isn't," she corrected. "I still think you were in either stage one or two of physician burnout back then. And I think that whatever's going on with you got worse after Lori's daughter died. I watched you at the memorial, and you looked like you were carrying the show for the family. That wears on you. You can only handle so much, and it's not because you're a mental midget. It's because you're human.

"You have to be careful, Marybeth. The third stage is chronic stress, and the fourth stage is burnout crisis."

"So, you think I'm suffering from physician burnout brought on by all the psychological trauma? Are you saying it's all in my head?"

Dr. Reed laughed. "No, it's not in your head. It's in your adrenal glands. Chronic stress takes its toll, and your adrenal glands respond. They start to shut down, and the symptoms get a lot worse in a short time. Let's do a workup on your fatigue and rule out any other medical reasons first. If everything else is normal, we'll investigate adrenal fatigue."

First and foremost, Dr. Reed assured me that my symptoms weren't abnormal. Fatigue always had a subtle start: a pervasive, nagging lack of energy. Lots of women in their late forties and early fifties experienced profound fatigue. There were many different reasons for it, which is why the

A busy life can cause you to be tired, but it doesn't cause the overwhelming fatigue I experienced.

medical workup was extensive. A busy life can cause you to be tired, but it doesn't cause the overwhelming fatigue I experienced. There had to be something more to it.

Other than hormones, depression, and living a ridiculously busy life, other medical reasons for fatigue include:

- **Anemia:** This is a prevalent cause of fatigue in women. You may have heavy periods that are longer than usual, which causes anemia. A simple CBC (complete blood count) can screen for anemia. Anemia can be the result of iron deficiency, decreased folic acid, or inadequate vitamin B12. You can also have anemia due to blood in your stool or urine or other forms of blood loss. Your CBC and a guaiac test (detects blood in stool) can help identify causes of anemia. If you are fifty or older, you should have already had a colonoscopy. If you haven't, get one.

- **Thyroid disease:** An overactive or underactive thyroid can cause fatigue. Hypothyroidism causes weight gain, cold intolerance, hair loss, joint pain, constipation, menstrual irregularity, and fatigue. Hyperthyroidism can cause agitation, a racing pulse, heat intolerance, and weight loss at first, but as your thyroid "burns out," you may complain of fatigue and weight gain. The best test to evaluate your thyroid is TSH level. TSH levels measure how much thyroid hormone the brain receives that is unbound, and it's more reliable than a simple T4 level.

- **Menopause:** Most of us are aware of the ravages of menopause—another topic our mothers didn't discuss with us. Symptoms include irregular to absent periods, hot flashes, night sweats, insomnia or restlessness, moodiness, inability to concentrate, and, yes, fatigue. A simple Follicle Stimulating Hormone test (FSH) can tell you if you're in menopause, but it can't tell you if you are in that lovely perimenopausal time of life.

- **Autoimmune diseases:** Unfortunately, a lot of autoimmune diseases can appear in your forties and fifties. A few common ones include lupus, rheumatoid arthritis, ankylosing spondylitis, and fibromyalgia. These unwelcome guests cause fatigue coupled with muscle and joint pain, skin rashes, and emotional lability. If you're having muscle and joint pain that seems to travel around your body in no apparent pattern, you may have an autoimmune disease. Your doctor can order a basic rheumatoid panel, including an Anti-Nuclear Antibodies (ANA) and sed rate, which help diagnose your issues. If these are positive, seek the help of a rheumatologist who specializes in these types of diseases.

- **Infections:** Most of us recognize acute bacterial or viral infections because their symptoms are readily apparent. Symptoms may include fatigue, chills, fever, nausea, and vomiting. Chronic infections can be insidious, and many viral infections have a post-viral syndrome that persists for weeks to months after the acute infection is gone. Talk to your doctor about screening for viral conditions such as COVID-19, mononucleosis, hepatitis, HIV, and cytomegalovirus. Persistent fatigue after an acute infection may be the ordinary course of the disease, but don't ignore your symptoms.

- **Other illnesses:** This list is endless, but here are a few where fatigue is a pervasive symptom: high blood pressure, diabetes, heart disease, kidney disease, multiple sclerosis, adrenal insufficiency, and cancer.

Another common cause of overwhelming fatigue is depression. Depression doesn't discriminate based on education level, socioeconomic status, or marital status. Almost 30 percent of women will experience some form of depression or anxiety disorder during their lifetime.

I'm not a psychiatrist, but I do know there's a difference between actual clinical depression and a normal response to a stressful life. People often experience the symptoms of depression from being under extreme pressure. Usually, we recognize the cause of our funk, fix it (or live through it), and then get back to normal. This funk isn't depression; it's life. So, if you know you're going through a horrendously stressful time, you're profoundly tired, have gained a few extra pounds, and can't concentrate or sleep, you're probably not depressed. You're having a normal response to a dysphoric phase of life.

Dr. Reed and I determined that I was in this category. Not depressed, only going through a roller coaster of crazy. I kept falling down, but I always got back up. She did, however, remind me to check in with my therapist if the episodes of sadness became more profound.

In contrast, here are the symptoms of major depression:

Group 1:
- Sad or irritable mood
- Loss of interest/capacity for pleasure

Group 2:
- Sleep problems (too much or too little)

- Impaired decision-making
- Lack of concentration
- Changes in appetite
- Suicidal thoughts (especially planning it)
- A feeling of guilt, worthlessness, or self-blame
- Profound fatigue levels
- Psychomotor agitation/retardation (fidgeting relentlessly or always slouching)

To be diagnosed with major depression, a person must have one symptom from group one and four symptoms from group two.

You might be thinking that everyone you know may be depressed because they suffer from some of these symptoms. The difference between clinical depression and situational depression is the duration and severity of symptoms—how they negatively impact your daily life.

If your score reveals that you're suffering from major depression, stop reading this book and call your doctor right now! Help is only a phone call away.

If you scored a little higher on the depression scale than you thought you would, you aren't alone. You're probably closer to normal than you think. Mild to moderate depression is often a companion to an intense lifestyle.

You can't become majorly depressed overnight, so stay ahead of it. You should take any symptoms

> *If your score reveals that you're suffering from major depression, stop reading this book and call your doctor right now! Help is only a phone call away.*

of depression seriously. I've watched many of my patients spiral from a minor depression into a significant depression. Depression kills. The suicide rate for women forty-five to sixty-four years old rose more than 50 percent from 2000 to 2018.

Please seek help—even if you think you may be only mildly depressed. Your doctor can help you sort it out. Start with your family physician, internist, or OB/GYN. They can talk through your symptoms and refer you to a psychologist or psychiatrist if needed.

Depression is caused by a chemical imbalance in the brain. Serotonin and dopamine—the two major mood chemicals—can get out of balance and cause you to be depressed. Stress can cause depression, and chronic stress can cause these chemicals to become progressively unbalanced, which spirals you from minor depression to major depression if left untreated. Taking antidepressants when you have a minor depression isn't a sign of weakness; it's a sign that you're taking care of yourself.

If your medical workup for fatigue showed no medical reasons for being so tired, or you and your doctor have determined that you aren't depressed, then it's time to consider Superwoman Syndrome.

A gallon of blood tests, an EKG, and some hormone levels later determined that I wasn't in menopause, my thyroid was fine, and I wasn't clinically depressed. I was suffering from adrenal fatigue.

Adrenal fatigue isn't the same as adrenal insufficiency, which is an autoimmune disorder. Adrenal fatigue means that the stress hormone levels are so chronically high that your adrenals are tired and telling you to eff off!

I quickly skipped through the third stage of burnout—chronic stress in the months and early years after Elise's death. Stage four was burnout crisis. This is when stress kills, and after the myriad of medical tests, it's exactly where my doctor said I was.

Many physicians argue that adrenal fatigue doesn't exist. They think the symptoms attributed to this disorder are vague and can be explained by other

Adrenal fatigue isn't the same as adrenal insufficiency, which is an autoimmune disorder.

medical conditions if you look hard enough. The Endocrine Society, the world's largest organization of endocrinologists—people who research and treat patients with diseases related to glands and hormones—flatly says that adrenal fatigue isn't a real disease. They encourage a complete workup like I underwent to rule out any other medical issues that can cause the fatigue.

There are two different kinds of stress: acute and chronic. Acute stress is short-lived. You feel it when you're holding the steering wheel and almost collide with another vehicle or when a wild animal is chasing you. It helps you escape a dangerous experience or do something fun and exhilarating like skydiving. It's not usually harmful and vanishes when the situation is over.

Chronic stress lingers over time. The triggers that cause the stress response are persistent, and your body is constantly releasing stress hormones like cortisol and epinephrine. This kind of stress strains the adrenal glands, which invariably leaves them incapable of meeting the body's demands. Chronic stress is the most common cause of adrenal fatigue and burnout.

Adrenal fatigue is diagnosed with either a DUTCH test (dried urine test for comprehensive hormones) or a saliva cortisol test. I did the saliva test. The test involves spitting into a test tube over a twenty-four-hour period. Cortisol is measured four times—8:00 a.m., noon, 4:00 p.m., and between 11:00 p.m. and midnight. This test showed that I had almost no cortisol and a lower-than-normal progesterone level.

Chronic stress is the most common cause of adrenal fatigue and burnout.

In 2019, the World Health Organization (WHO) recognized Burnout Syndrome as an occupational phenomenon, stressing that this is not a medical condition but a syndrome resulting from chronic workplace stress that hasn't been successfully managed. I disagree and argue that it *becomes* a medical condition as it progresses toward chronic burnout.

The WHO defines Burnout Syndrome as:

- Feelings of excessive energy depletion and fatigue
- Increased mental distance from one's job
- Feelings of negativity or cynicism toward one's job
- Reduced professional efficacy

The WHO also estimates that between 32 percent and 60 percent of medical professionals suffer from Burnout Syndrome due to excessive workloads and high patient expectations. More women doctors are affected due to the compounding effect of home stress piled upon work stress.

For me, adrenal fatigue was a genuine medical disorder. My doctor had tried to find another cause, but at a time in my life when my cortisol levels should have been rising due to perimenopause, my cortisol levels were almost nonexistent. As I tried to be Superwoman, block out my grief, and be everything for everybody, the stress was killing me. It had exhausted my adrenal glands, depleted my ability to maintain my cortisol levels, and caused my extreme fatigue and a myriad of other symptoms.

Adrenal Fatigue—now I had a name for what was wrong with me. Dr. Reed gave me some sound medical advice, and I went to work on fixing myself.

"I'm glad you finally went to the doctor," Lori said. "I never realized that stress could build up and make you sick like that. What's the next step to getting back to your normal self?"

"I honestly don't think I'm ever going to go back to my normal self," I said. "According to Dr. Reed, *my* normal isn't normal, and that's what's killing me. I have some hard choices to make."

"Welcome to my world," Lori said. "My life will never be normal without my daughter. I miss her every day."

"I miss the smile on your face, my friend," I quietly replied. "We both have some work to do on ourselves, and sadly, it can't be a collaborative effort. We can't fix each other, and we can't go back in time to change things. We have to figure out how to live with the grief and trauma, some of which was self-induced in my case."

"Let me know when you figure it out," Lori said with a sigh.

3

I CAN'T SLEEP

Sleep disruption is one of the most pervasive symptoms of adrenal fatigue caused by Superwoman Syndrome. Lack of restful sleep—or sleep deprivation—can lead to increased appetite, which leads to eating carbs and sugars to stay awake during the day, which leads to weight gain, which leads to further stress about weight gain. Then you throw in a psychotic schedule, which fosters a poor wake-sleep pattern, which begins with caffeine overload in the morning and ends with alcohol consumption to make you sleepy before bed. This unhealthy pattern of mine was a recipe for disaster.

Art, my new husband, gently nudged my shoulder to wake me up. "Honey, it looks like you spent half the night on the couch again. Was I snoring?"

"No. I woke up at two and couldn't go back to sleep. Too much brain activity. I couldn't shut it off. I kept going over my to-do list and couldn't figure out how I was going to get it all done," I answered while yawning and getting up off the couch.

"You need to stop thinking so much. Although, I'm surprised you could think at all after drinking almost a whole bottle of wine after dinner."

"I didn't drink the whole bottle. I was just trying to quiet the noise," I replied sheepishly.

"We need to figure out how to get you to shut your brain off and get some real sleep without drinking. Not a good habit to get into," Art said.

The best, first thing you can do to recover from adrenal fatigue is to normalize your sleep pattern. My wake-sleep pattern started with a gallon of caffeine in the morning and ended with a gallon of wine at night. Then I'd wake up multiple times in the night and stare at the ceiling, wondering why I couldn't sleep.

Most adults need seven to eight hours of quality sleep on a regular basis every night. Yes, on a regular basis. But that's not what we do in our overscheduled American lifestyle. And this insane pattern starts with our youth. For example, Caitlin had to be at cross-country practice at 5:45 a.m. During her freshman and sophomore years, I got up at 5:00 a.m., took her to practice, got my run in, then got her sister breakfasted and ready for the bus by 7:00 a.m. I liked to go to bed at 9:00 p.m., but that rarely happened. That pattern had to change. It was time to take sleep more seriously.

Why is sleep important?

There are so many benefits of good sleep habits. You have a better immune system, so you get sick less often. Sleep helps us maintain a healthy weight, and you feel less hungry when you're well rested. It also decreases your risk for chronic diseases

> *The best, first thing you can do to recover from adrenal fatigue is to normalize your sleep pattern.*

like diabetes and heart disease. Adequate sleep reduces stress, improves mood, and allows us to think more clearly. Healthy sleep patterns lead to more quality work, less crankiness, and making more logical decisions. These are all good things, and definitely, many of these things are awry when you suffer from adrenal fatigue.

So, why can't we sleep?

There are many causes of sleep disorders. Sleep impediments can include stress, anxiety, chronic pain, heartburn, asthma, side effects of medication, too much caffeine or alcohol, and sleep apnea. According to the CDC, 35 percent of all adults report that they get less than seven hours of sleep. There's no difference in this number between men and women. That's a lot of tired people, and in fact, I bet the numbers are worse than reported.

So, how can you improve your sleep? You must change your routine.

- Exercise earlier in the day.
- Have a very comfortable bed, soft sheets, and the perfect pillow.
- Make your room dark, cold, and quiet.
- Play background white noise.
- Avoid caffeine four hours before your planned sleep.
- Avoid or reduce alcohol consumption within four hours of planned sleep. Many people wake up in the middle of the night when the sedative effect wears off.
- Avoid large meals and beverages late at night. They can cause heartburn and frequent middle-of-the-night bathroom trips.
- Avoid stimulants like allergy medication in the afternoon if possible.

- Relax before bed with yoga, stretching, a hot bath, or a good book.
- Avoid screen time two hours before bedtime. Cell phones, computers, and televisions emit a blue light that can interrupt your circadian rhythm.

If you've changed your routine and are still having sleep pattern issues, call your doctor to discuss common sleep disorders.

Signs of a sleep disorders include:

- Frequent, loud snoring
- Pauses in breathing during sleep
- Trouble waking up in the morning even though you had adequate time to sleep
- Difficulty staying awake during the day
- Frequent waking in the middle of the night
- Restless legs or painful, itchy burning in your legs at night that feels better with massage (also known as restless leg syndrome)

We are a nation of sleepyheads. We all need more rest. Adults who are short sleepers tend to have significantly more health issues than similar people who get enough rest. Sleepy people are also cranky, have difficulty making good decisions, and often don't play nice with others. I was one definitely of them! After being diagnosed with adrenal fatigue, my doctor recommended that I start taking my sleep

After being diagnosed with adrenal fatigue, my doctor recommended that I start taking my sleep seriously.

seriously. She thought that normalized sleep patterns improved adrenal fatigue more than almost any other intervention.

I did a few essential things:

- I had a long discussion with my teenage daughters about my need to get better sleep. We also discussed how their health would improve if they had a better sleep pattern.
- I started going to bed at 9:00 p.m., or as close as I could. I got up at 5:30 a.m. to get my routine started.
- I started taking a hormone supplement an hour before bedtime to help with my low progesterone level. It helped me get to sleep without sleeping pills or wine.
- Instead of coffee, I started my day with an Athletics Greens shake, sixteen ounces of cold water, and exercise. Early morning exercise is better than coffee to wake up your system. I can't say I completely cut out caffeine. Instead, I reduced my intake to one cup of coffee in the morning after my exercise.
- I turned off the ringer on my phone and silenced all social media notifications after dinner. No more late-night TV unless it was a significant sporting event, which was an exception. I got in bed with a magazine or a good book.
- If I had a glass of wine, only one was acceptable, and it had to be earlier in the evening.
- On incredibly busy days, which there were a few, meditation helped center my mind and get ready for sleep.
- I bought a ridiculously expensive Westin Heavenly Bed, which is the most comfortable bed in the world. Worth the money! Cool sheets and a slightly cooler temperature for sleeping also helped.

- I embraced naps. Not every day, but on the days I worked from home. On Tuesdays, Fridays, and weekends, I welcomed a short catnap of twenty to thirty minutes after lunch. The small nap refreshed me.

My sleeping pattern normalized quite a bit by making these little tweaks. I encourage you to troubleshoot your sleep patterns. It will help with your decision-making, weight control, and overall health. Get better sleep. You and the people around you will thank me for it.

I'M GAINING WEIGHT

"Do you think I'm getting fat?" I asked my husband.

Art gave me an "Are you kidding me?" look.

"Of course not, honey, you're just a little softer than you've been in the past. So am I." He rolled his beautiful blue but not so sympathetic eyes. "You're still beautiful, even in a potato sack."

"You don't like this dress?" Heck, I wasn't too fond of the dress myself, but my choices were sparse.

"You have much nicer, babe," he replied.

"Not that fit," I snapped back. I took off the basic, black shift dress and dove into my closet to search for another option.

It was Friday night—date night. The girls usually stayed at their grandmother's every Friday night so that we could get a break from the family chaos. It was a little chilly out, and I was tired. I was always tired. My closet was in disarray, a rainbow pile of dresses strewn on the floor. I couldn't find anything to wear out to dinner. I came out in another simple black dress, feeling like a cow. It was only a little tight, so I could make it work.

"When did I start getting soft?" I asked.

I could tell from the look in Art's eyes that he didn't want to have this conversation.

Taking a longer than needed deep breath, he answered, "Well, babe, probably about the same time you stopped running. You know you haven't run very much lately."

He was right. I couldn't find the motivation to run or exercise at all anymore.

"And we don't eat dinner together most days because of my shift," he continued, "So I have no idea what you eat."

Again, he was right. We didn't eat dinner together because he worked from 1:00 p.m. to 9:00 p.m. I often scraped something together for the girls and ate whatever was left in the refrigerator—or didn't eat at all. A bag of potato chips and a glass of wine was a decent dinner on a school night.

"I guess you're right. I need to get my act together." I thought to myself, *I feel fat, and my new husband seems to agree with me, so I guess that means I'm fat.*

As if he could read my mind, Art interjected, "And don't complain about being fat to anyone outside this house. You're likely to get punched."

Duly noted, I thought.

To put things into context, I've always been thin. When I graduated from high school, I weighed ninety-five pounds and wore a double zero petite. Throughout college, medical school, and into my early marriage, I gained about ten pounds. So, a little over a hundred pounds was my average weight, and that's where I was comfortable. Four pregnancies and twenty-five years later, I was still sitting right around a hundred or so. I'm five foot two and very small-boned, so I wasn't considered underweight.

Honestly, I liked being thin. I worked hard to be thin. I probably was egotistical about being considered skinny. And if I ever noticed that my pants were getting a little tight, all I had to do was increase my exercise routine and be more mindful about what I ate, and those few pounds always disappeared. After my first pregnancy, I ran my first marathon to lose weight, then went on to run dozens more. I ran a marathon when pregnant with my second daughter. After my fourth pregnancy, I took on the challenge of an Ironman Triathlon, and the weight disappeared.

Throughout the years, I realized I was blessed with a fast metabolism and could eat almost anything. Until I couldn't. In my early forties, I noticed it was harder and harder to stay thin. It wasn't even the weight; it was how I felt in my clothes. I felt bloated and uncomfortable. I started buying size zero, then size two. It was when the size two felt tight that I got concerned. My weight gain prompted another visit to my doctor.

"So, Dr. Reed, am I going through menopause, and this is one of the side effects? Do most middle-aged women end up looking like a potato?" I asked her.

"No, you aren't going through menopause yet, but you may be experiencing perimenopausal symptoms," she answered.

"Are you sure?" I reiterated.

She sat down on the leather exam stool, put the chart on the counter with a thump, turned to look at me, and said, "You're not fat! You're a little more normal like the rest of us instead of being that uber-fit athlete you're used to being."

I could see the laughter in her eyes. I was sure she was thinking, *Finally*! She'd heard me whine about being fat before, but it was always shortly after giving birth.

"How's your fatigue?" she inquired, changing gears.

"Not much better yet, but I'm trying to work on my stress level," I answered, knowing I was lying. Nothing was getting much better. Ignoring the problem wasn't working.

I had to admit that my weight gain wasn't only the lack of cortisol; it was poor habits that I'd fallen into because of my busy life. Didn't everybody graze their children's leftovers instead of eating a real dinner because they're trying to multitask? Probably not! On a typical weeknight, I'd come home from work, either heat something or cook dinner, chuck it at the kids, put in a load of laundry, wash the dishes, get on a conference call, and then eat whatever was left. It didn't help that Caitlin ran about fifty miles a week and could eat an entire pound of pasta in one sitting, and Sasha was a horrendously picky eater. It was also unreasonable to think that I'd cook an entirely different meal for myself; who had time for that? If I added the amount of alcohol I drank to relieve the crazy, I'd created a recipe for belly fat. Yep, for the first time in my life, I had a pooch, and I wasn't too fond of it.

"If you get your stress under control, you'll lose weight," Dr. Reed told me.

She was right. It was time to get this under control before I became a real cow. By the time I left her office, I had realized that no one else could do this for me. I needed to get serious about my diet and exercise habits. It was clear that it wasn't going to fix itself.

"If you get your stress under control, you'll lose weight," Dr. Reed told me.

The hormonal changes of perimenopause make you more likely to gain weight around your abdomen than around your hips and thighs—thus the aforementioned pooch. On top of that, muscle mass decreases with age—3 percent to 8 percent per decade after age thirty. Muscle mass loss slows down your metabolism, and if you continue to eat as you always have and don't increase your physical activity, you're going to gain weight. It's a simple formula. You need about two hundred calories less per day in your fifties than you needed in your thirties. Add the increased stress in life that causes elevated levels of a hormone called ghrelin, which makes you hungrier. Your body thinks it needs more fuel due to the increased stress, so you're hungry. And the lack of adequate sleep makes you feel hungrier—a wretched feedback loop for someone who complained of weight gain.

So, what's the magic formula to reverse this process? It's pretty simple. Mindfulness. It would help you to be mindful of better sleep patterns, decreased stress, eating less and eating healthier, consuming less alcohol, and moving more with added strength training.

Here are some changes that can help you get back on track:

- Pay attention to what you're eating and drinking.
- Start with a vegan cleanse. You can do a three- to five-day juice cleanse if you like. I prefer a three-day cleanse of mixed raw and cooked vegetables, flaxseed granola, and no alcohol. The combination cleans out my system (literally) and gets me started in the right direction. I follow the cleanse from *The Metabolism Plan* by Lyn-Genet Recitas.
- A plant-based diet, modified paleo, or a Mediterranean diet are the healthiest options. I'm not a fan of keto, but some people find that helpful. You don't have to go nuts and change all your habits at once, but these types of diets help balance your gut health and improve hormone regulation.
- Replace butter or margarine with olive oil or avocado oil.

- Eat lean meats in smaller portions, or substitute healthy protein from soy, quinoa, eggs, dairy, nuts, seeds, and beans.

- Eat a mixture of raw and cooked vegetables, which helps to fill you up and aids in digestion. Make your plate as colorful as it can be, and be sure that it's more than half vegetables.

- Cut out soft drinks. Even diet drinks are bad because they alter your stomach's pH and make your body crave sugar.

- Plan and regulate your alcohol consumption or quit drinking altogether.

- Drink half your body weight in ounces of water every day to stay well hydrated. This also helps to curb hunger. I start my day by drinking a sixteen-ounce glass of cold water. Cold water kickstarts your metabolism because your body has to use calories to heat the water. Remember that your brain actually can't tell the difference between being thirsty and hungry, so take care of the thirst to decrease your hunger drive. Take a bottle of water with you whenever you leave your house.

- Use a smaller plate and sit down to eat. This helps to regulate portion size.

- Eat slower and take smaller bites. The act of chewing makes you feel full faster.

- Stop grazing your kids' food. Make an appointment with yourself to eat dinner instead of shopping in the refrigerator.

- Plan your meals and shop on Saturday, followed by meal prep for the entire week on Sunday. This makes a huge difference, especially when your week goes wheels-off crazy.

- Never grocery shop when you're hungry. Somehow, those salty or sugary extras end up in the basket every time!
- Take-out food is forbidden unless it's an emergency! Hidden fats and sodium are everywhere.
- When you do eat out, split the meal with your spouse or take half of it home. Portion sizes are out of control in most restaurants, and if you plan, you won't feel the need to eat it all.

The bottom line is that you have to control your eating habits better as you age. You have to be mindful of your toxic habits. Make stress-induced eating a thing of the past. Proper hydration, portion control, and decreasing carbohydrates help to regulate your weight.

5

I'M DRINKING TOO MUCH

"Mom!" yelled Caitlin. "Why do you drink so much?"
Good question, I thought to myself, especially
from a fifteen-year-old. Caitlin was working on
a school project and wandered down to my room to ask for
some help. She found me fully clothed and asleep in my bed at
8:00 p.m. There was a half-full wine glass on my nightstand—
right where I left it. The bottle was in the kitchen, inside the
refrigerator door, empty. *I couldn't have drunk it all if I put
it back in the fridge. Someone else must have finished it.* My
husband was working late, so that argument didn't quite
stand up.

It was a typical Tuesday night in my household.

Earlier that evening, after a long day of patients and an
argument with one of the other doctors, and I had a glass of wine
while cooking dinner. Then, while sipping on the second glass, I
helped Sasha with her homework. I wasn't even sure I ate a real
dinner; probably grazed on what was left on Sasha's plate since
she never ate it all. The third glass was after yelling at Sasha to

take a shower and get ready for bed. I'm not sure when I poured the fourth glass.

"I don't drink that much. It's been a rough day," I replied, shaking myself awake and trying to sound coherent.

"I don't know, Mom. I know that Lori is worried about you."

"Lori has enough to worry about, and I don't think I drink much more than most of your friends' moms," I said, starting to get annoyed. "Why are you talking to Lori about my drinking?"

"She still checks in with me, and it came up in conversation when I told her about Sarah's mom getting out of the drunk tank."

"What?" I was fully awake now.

"She was supposedly depressed and drinking all day when Sarah was at school. She ended up in the hospital with some stomach issues, according to Sarah. I told Lori about how tired you've been and how you drink to go to sleep."

"I love that you're concerned about me, but I don't drink that much. Things have been very stressful lately," I said in a sad voice. Another stellar Mom moment.

"I'll call Sarah's mom tomorrow and see if she's okay," I continued. "I'm going back to bed, this time with PJs on. I love you."

"Love you too, Mom. And don't worry, I don't think you're a drunk. But maybe you should drink less?"

Later, when I was sober, it occurred to me that somehow in our neighborhood, habitual drinking, especially for middle-aged women, had become the norm. I wasn't alone. When I was troubleshooting my sleep problems, the first thing that came up was that I started my day with a bucket of caffeine and ended my day with wine. I belonged to three wine clubs and had at least one drink every day.

For over twenty years, I'd been running with two other women in their late forties-early fifties who had stressful jobs, had also gone through divorces, and had issues with their older children. Very similar lives. Our Saturday morning runs were often group therapy sessions. I'd met my new husband in this running group. We allowed a few men to join us from time to time to look social.

"Alice, what's up with you this morning?" I inquired as I laced up my running shoes. "You look like a truck ran over you. Didn't you sleep well last night?"

"I'm okay. I just had a few too many glasses of wine last night," she replied. "I have a teensy-weensy hangover, but I'll be okay. Six o'clock came early. I made sure I drank a gallon of water when I got up this morning."

We were all training for the Dallas marathon, so ten miles around the lake was on the schedule.

"The best cure I know for a hangover is a ten-mile run. It'll make you sweat it out," I said with a laugh. If I was honest, I had a bit of a hangover as well.

"Do you think we drink too much?" Alice asked the group.

Betty chimed in, "Doesn't everyone have a glass of wine to go to bed at night?"

"Yes," we all answered almost simultaneously.

"And sometimes, it's not only one," Alice muttered. "In fact, it's almost the whole bottle several times a week. Maybe we all have a problem."

"No, I don't think so," I replied. "It's not like we drink to wake ourselves up in the morning. We don't drink before work or at lunch, and I don't know about you guys, but I don't crave it during the day. We must be okay. Group therapy session over, let's get to the run."

In the back of my mind, I knew my habitual drinking was not okay.

Did most American women drink three bottles of wine a week? It turned out the answer was no. But in my small Texas town, this was the norm. We lived in an affluent community full of stressed-out women who felt the pressure of keeping up with the Joneses and Superwoman Syndrome. You were either a stay-at-home mom whose kid was so overscheduled it was ridiculous, and you felt the stress of trying to have the perfect home and the ideal child while maintaining your marriage, or you felt the pressure of trying to do all that *and* maintain a professional job or business. It made for a community of alcohol-dependent women.

In the back of my mind, I knew my habitual drinking was not okay.

We weren't unusual. The use of alcohol to mitigate stress is a worldwide phenomenon amongst professional women and affluent stay-at-home moms. These stay-at-home supermoms have a different version of Superwoman Syndrome, but the pressure is still there. In the United States, 30 percent of adults admit to abusing alcohol at some point in their lives, and 15 percent are confirmed alcoholics. In my non-scientific research, I believe alcoholism is probably a lot higher than is cited.

But we weren't alcoholics; we were only habitual drinkers. That wasn't the same thing. Or was it? Were we alcohol dependent or alcohol-addicted? It was a question we each would have to answer independently.

So, what's the difference? According to the National Institute on Alcohol Abuse and Alcoholism (NIAAA), excessive drinking or binge drinking is defined as drinking more than four drinks in two hours for women or five drinks in two hours for men. It can also be defined as more than eight drinks a week for women or ten drinks a week for men. The difference is that people who binge drink are usually drinking to get drunk. Conversely, alcoholics tend to have an almost everyday drinking habit and viscerally crave alcohol.

The Centers for Disease Control and Prevention (CDC) defines alcoholism as a dependency on alcohol. People with alcoholism have an intense craving and continue to drink even when doing so causes them physical and social problems. They consume alcohol almost daily and can't stop without help. Long-term alcohol abuse can change the chemical signaling in the brain, and without alcohol, people with alcoholism can experience seizures when trying to stop.

Men and women differ in their ability to metabolize alcohol. That glass of wine will go straight to your head, but not your husband's. Women get drunk much faster than men because men have a highly active form of alcohol dehydrogenase (ADH), the enzyme responsible for metabolizing alcohol in the stomach and liver. Women have almost no ADH in their stomachs, so we absorb the alcohol faster—more than 30 percent faster—over the same time period. Women also have a less active form of ADH in their liver, so our blood alcohol concentration (BAC) is significantly higher than men drinking the same amount. Women get drunk a lot faster than men.

Perhaps it's time to take a long, hard look at your drinking patterns. Let's break this down. Why do we drink? We drink to medicate our anxiety. We drink to decrease stress. We drink because it's socially acceptable. We drink because it's part of our entertainment. We drink because we're playing golf, where day drinking is entirely acceptable, even on a Tuesday. We drink because our kids are driving us bonkers. We drink because our husbands are never home. We drink because our employees are problematic. We drink because we don't know what to do next. We drink because we can't sleep. We drink because we're hungry but don't want to cook. We drink because it seems to be the answer to most of our problems.

Here's the crux of the problem: social drinking is one thing; habitually turning to alcohol is another. It's okay to be at a dinner party and have a glass of water or sparkling water with a lime in it, so it looks like it's a gin and tonic. No one seems to notice. I can't remember the last time someone asked me what was in my glass.

> *Here's the crux of the problem: social drinking is one thing; habitually turning to alcohol is another.*

Caitlin was fifteen years old when she started observing that I drank too much. After Elise passed away, it was obvious that I was drinking more. I had to look myself in the mirror and decide if I had a problem or if it was something I could control. Was it a bad habit, or was it an addiction? I knew the answer would be to either completely stop drinking or learn how to manage it.

Experts say you should totally abstain from drinking, which will take care of the problem. But doing that felt like throwing in the towel and saying I couldn't control it. I had to find out if I could manage my drinking. I liked wine. I enjoyed my wine clubs. I had an excellent wine refrigerator and didn't want to give it up. But my relationship with alcohol had to change. Instead of being my stress reliever, it had become one of my stressors.

Alcohol alters your sleep patterns, and not for good. It also doesn't help when you start your day with a fuzzy brain. So how did I change my relationship with alcohol but not give it up completely? You can cognitively decide when it's okay to drink. Yes, you can plan when you drink. You have to do it ahead of time because, after that second glass of wine, the third and the fourth and the fifth are very easy to pour since you are cognitively impaired. You have to decide it's okay to pour one glass, even two, on a Friday night and then put it away. You can decide that you're not drinking on days that start with T or only drinking on days that begin with S. They even make smaller bottles that only have two glasses of wine in them. Your rule can be to drink only one of those small bottles. Another useful trick is to have a glass of water in between each drink, so you're drinking less alcohol over an extended period. Portion control is critical. You have to measure what goes in your wine glass or mixed drink. No more free pouring! A glass of wine is five ounces, and a mixed drink gets only one shot!

Use a smaller glass or mix your wine with sparkling water or club soda and make a wine spritzer. That way, your wine lasts longer. I also recommend giving up any hard liquor with fruity mixers that tend to taste like punch—it's too easy to drink too much without realizing it. They also have lots of sugar in them and can be part of your weight problem. Stick to things you can count.

Remember, this isn't willpower. You decide that you control your body, not the alcohol. Stop overdrinking.

It is not an easy task to control or plan your drinking. Many people cannot plan when they drink, cannot stop with one drink, constantly crave alcohol, and the alcohol is toxic to their bodies. This is the definition of a real addiction, not a bad habit, and it's time to reach out for help to quit. Remember the difference between heavy or binge drinking and alcoholism. Do you crave alcohol? Do you fail every time you try to plan your drinking? If this is you, many community resources can help you, and I encourage you to reach out to a therapist to help you navigate your recovery. You can do it, but you don't have to be a martyr. Ask for help.

It is not an easy task to control or plan your drinking.

Need any more incentive to get your drinking under control? Let's talk about the effect of alcohol on your blood sugar levels. When alcohol enters your bloodstream, your body's top priority is to get rid of it as quickly as possible. To clear your bloodstream of alcohol, your body shifts resources away from other processes. Alcohol stimulates the secretion of insulin, which over time can cause insulin resistance and even diabetes. An estimated 45 to 70 percent of alcoholics suffer from liver disease, insulin resistance, or diabetes.

Furthermore, there is the psychological effect. I turned to alcohol as a stress reliever. Then it became a stressor. Why? Because while drinking seems uplifting at first, the toxicity of the alcohol quickly takes hold. Prolonged drinking eventually causes levels of happiness-inducing neurotransmitters, namely serotonin and dopamine, to plummet. The result is an inability to enjoy activities, feelings of hopelessness, a lack of motivation, guilt, anger, and frustration. You're drinking to medicate your anxiety, but prolonged drinking increases anxiety and its accompanying depression the more protracted the drinking continues.

We need to find better ways to deal with our stress. I turned to meditation, yoga, and a gratitude journal. I also reached out to a therapist to talk through the grief and anxiety roller coaster I lived for more than twenty years. It helped. I recommend having someone to talk to outside of your family. Your confidant may be a therapist, counselor, minister, or even a long-term friend who lives in another state.

Caitlin became my accountability partner, with Art as a backup when she was away at college. She knows it is okay to call me out if she thinks I've had too much or am falling back into the old pattern. Art feels very comfortable handing me a glass of water. I plan my drinking and try to keep it social. Alcohol isn't my stress reliever anymore.

Many women trying to maintain sanity with a hectic, stressful lifestyle are overwhelmed by their daily lives. We need to find healthier ways to mitigate stress and realize it is misguided to see alcohol as a stress management tool. If you can't learn to plan when you drink, stop overdrinking, and make it more social, then it's time to quit.

6

I DON'T WANT TO EXERCISE

t was 5:30 a.m., and all was quiet in the house. My alarm went off, and it was time to run. I hit the snooze button and curled up with my fantastic pillow. It was so soft and cuddly, and I was warm and cozy. Perhaps I could savor the moment and snuggle with Art. He barely moved as I cuddled against him, and the dog snuggled between us. My running shoes could wait. I was savoring my quiet time, and I deserved it. This early morning time was the only respite from the chaos that I had. I hit the snooze button again. I didn't feel like running today. Lately, I didn't ever feel like running. Even if I pried myself from my bed, I often wandered into the kitchen, savored my coffee, walked the dog a block or so, and made every excuse for why I didn't have time or energy, or it was too hot or too cold. Running wasn't essential anymore. I wasn't sure when that had happened.

Running has always been at the center of my life. It was my happy place. I started running in the fifth grade because I couldn't hit, kick, or catch a ball. And I was good at it! My first race was a 5K on July 4, 1979. I won my age group, and my running career started. I ran in high school, college, and beyond. Even during medical school, when time was so precious, I ran to clear my head and keep the pounds off. After having my first daughter, I ran my first marathon to take off the baby weight. I figured training for a marathon would help me build my fledgling practice and help me get back in shape. A win-win proposal. I ran a marathon while pregnant with Caitlin and then qualified for Boston the next year. I made the front page of the local paper's sports section, which was great free advertising for my growing sports medicine practice. I ate, breathed, lived, and talked about distance running all day long. My license plate even said RUNDOC.

Running helped me during the early years and saved my sanity during my divorce and beyond. My stress increased during my divorce, so I took it to another level, training for a full Ironman Triathlon—140.6 miles of swimming, cycling, and running. Two full Ironman Triathlon finishes taught me I could push through anything. This knowledge helped me transition into my next phase of life as a single, independent woman with three children and an ever-growing private practice.

Running had even brought Art and me together. We met on a Saturday morning run with my peeps at the lake. He decided he wanted to run with the "Fun Girls" after seeing how animated my friends and I were on our runs. He proposed a few years later after a typical Saturday morning run.

Running had always been an integral part of my life, but for some reason, it had now lost its appeal. Another stress reliever had become a stressor.

And I was reminded of it all the time. "What race are you training for?" asked my patients on a daily basis.

My last full marathon was Boston in 2014, the year after the bombing. The fatigue was starting to get real at that point but hadn't peaked. I was so tired that my time was over an hour longer than my previous attempt at the same race. Pathetic. My competitive personality took over, and I beat myself up internally for the slow time. It was embarrassing! If I couldn't be competitive, then why run?

> *If I couldn't be competitive, then why run?*

"Why can't you be happy that you finished?" asked Art. "Stop beating yourself up! Most women your age can't even think about finishing a Half Ironman! Stop it!"

I'd just finished Ironman 70.3 in Chattanooga and was crying at the finish line. After a very tough bike course, my time sucked, and I'd died an excruciating death during the half-marathon. I felt defeated.

"You don't understand!" I yelled back. "I suck!"

"You don't suck," he answered quickly. "You just haven't been training as much as usual, and you're getting a little older. It's normal to lose a step or two."

"I don't like it, and I feel like my body is betraying me," I replied with a little sniffle.

"I would still love you even if you walked the whole thing. I'm proud of you. Why can't you just be happy participating, my love?" Art gently asked as he placed a blanket around my shoulders and picked up my bike and gear bag.

Herein lies the problem. My perfectionist type-A personality, combined with my internal need to be the best, had derailed my athletic career. Why couldn't I be happy to participate? Why did I have to be on the podium all the time? When we got home from Tennessee, I hung my bike on the garage wall, and it didn't move for almost a year. I was done for now.

During this time, Caitlin was steadily improving her times in high school cross country and track. College coaches even scouted her. I was the consummate track

> *My perfectionist type-A personality, combined with my internal need to be the best, had derailed my athletic career.*

junkie mom. We talked about race strategy. We talked about her training. We talked about her nutrition and sleep. I was so excited for her and her progress. Watching her race made me remember what I loved about competitive distance running.

"Mom, Coach Leonard says I have to start running twice a day this summer to get my base fitness up for cross country. Can you wake me up at five-thirty every morning?" Caitlin asked at dinner one night. "And can you make sure I get out of bed?"

"Sure, honey. I'll set the alarm and make sure you're upright," I replied.

That short conversation put me back on the pavement in my running shoes. If I were going to get out of bed to wake Caitlin up, then why not lace up my own shoes?

At first, Caitlin ran with her friends, and I would jog in the neighborhood. Nothing big, only a few miles at a leisurely pace. And I took a lot of walk breaks. Then I started running with her during the summer before her senior year in high school. Slowly, I found it okay to jog. No races. No watch. Only the early morning silence and our heavy breathing. We didn't even need to talk. Those early morning jogs made me realize that even though I stopped racing, I was still a runner, and I missed it.

Art had been trying to convince me that I should be satisfied that I could run at all in my fifties. Lots of my friends and patients quit running some time ago because of back, hip, knee, or foot problems. Slowly, something changed in my attitude toward running. I no longer wanted to be hounded by it. I'm not sure if I'll ever train for a marathon again—maybe 2014 was my last—but the jury is still out.

I adopted a new attitude toward my fitness. I realized I'd been putting a lot of stress on myself by trying to run the times I had in my thirties. Even though when I closed my eyes, I thought I was twenty-five again, I needed to open my eyes and realize I was over fifty and should be happy to still be moving forward. I'd taken up triathlons in my forties to force me to cross-train because running every day was beating up my body. I now *participate* instead of *race*. I work out and run to be healthy and to mitigate stress—not to cause more!

Just because I wasn't racing anymore, it didn't mean I couldn't run, ride my bike, or go for a swim. So, I made a plan. I bought a Peloton bike, and that made cycling fun again. I found that mixing it up helped with my fatigue. Yoga, meditation, stretching, low-impact cycling, and long, slow runs all gave me the endorphins I craved, but none of them increased my stress hormones like racing or HIIT classes. Long, slow runs are now enjoyable and stress-free. I don't even wear a watch most of the time.

I was back with a new definition. Fit, fifty, and fabulous was my new motto. I was happy to participate, but with the competitive button on pause for now.

7

I DON'T FEEL SEXY

After my divorce, I was adamant that I'd never get married again. I felt like I had to take care of myself and my girls—a full-time job. Another man wasn't in the cards. Who had time for that? Of course, that was until I met Art.

Art was different. He was the consummate Boy Scout who would cross the street to help someone he didn't even know. He was a different kind of man. We met when he joined my running group to train for a marathon, even though our group was mainly made up of women. And then he stayed, joining us almost every week. He was relatively newly divorced and loved to tell us the details of his Internet dating. It was hilarious. Art was like one of the girls. Some other guys in the group came and went, but the core group of four women persisted for years. Art became number five, part of the band.

At some point, Art and I started to meet for dinner on Friday nights. The girls still went to their grandparents' house on Friday nights, which worked for everyone. They got Grandma time, and I could get up early on Saturday mornings to run without worrying about them. I hated eating alone on Fridays, so one weekend, I asked Art if he wanted to join me for dinner. As friends. Since he was often alone on Fridays, too, these dinners made sense. They were comfortable and easy. We talked about everything. No pressure. It was only a friend date. We friend-dated for over a year, until one night after a holiday party, I told him I didn't want to be his friend anymore. He had slowly seeped into my heart and softened it. He grew on me until I thought about him all the time.

Over the next year, our relationship deepened. Thanksgiving week in 2013, we went to Turks and Caicos for a holiday. Our exes had the kids, and it was the first time we'd spent that much time together. By the end of the week, I knew he was different—romantic, passionate, loving—not selfish, narcissistic, or demanding. He was a gentle, loving man. The kind I needed.

Almost a year later, he proposed to me after an eight-mile run. After a month of planning, he assembled my entire family, close friends, and even my staff to surprise me. It was an incredibly thoughtful and romantic gesture.

At the same place we'd met several years before, he asked, "Mary Elizabeth Crane, will you marry me?"

I replied quickly, "Of course I will!"

I had my Prince Charming. Fourteen months later, we had an incredibly romantic wedding on the beach in Kauai.

Yes, I did it; I got married again, and we were happy. Time passed, and the romance continued but naturally mellowed. As the chaos in our lives and my fatigue got worse, my libido slowly decreased. I liked sex, but I was never in the mood anymore. It's like exercise; once you lace up your running shoes and get out the door, you appreciate the runner's high from the endogenous opiates released by the run. Similarly, once you're in the throes of passion, I don't know anyone who doesn't enjoy a good orgasm. But like exercise, I had no desire to seek it out. I simply didn't feel like it.

"Baby, how about we go out for a nice dinner and then have a quiet adult evening tonight?" Art suggested.

The last thing I wanted to do was put on a dress and go out. I was exhausted, it was Friday, and it had been a hell of a week at the office.

As the chaos in our lives and my fatigue got worse, my libido slowly decreased.

Instead, I said, "Okay. We can drop Sasha at Grandma's on our way."

Art smiled. "I think that's a wonderful idea. A nice steak and a bottle of wine will make you relax after your stressful week."

In other words, he was thinking, *If I buy her a nice meal and ply her with wine, maybe I'll get lucky.*

We often went out on Friday nights for date night, which meant I'd put on nice clothes and ditch my yoga pants. Usually, we'd end the evening with a little romance between the sheets.

What had once been a weekly tradition now felt like a chore. I was faking it more and more. I made excuses for why we couldn't go out, and I felt increasingly guilty about how I was feeling. I loved Art and our relationship, but I didn't feel sexy or romantic. My clothes didn't fit well and made me feel even less attractive, but I had no desire to go shopping. I'd started wearing yoga pants and flannel PJs around the house and scrubs at work.

My fatigue made me cold all the time, so I started wearing flannel pajamas to bed. Sometimes, I'd wake up in the middle of the night naked and freezing because I'd had a hot flash and had unconsciously ripped off my PJs. Of course, when Art woke up in the morning and realized I was naked, he thought I did it on purpose to start something. That was the furthest thing from my mind, and it often led to hurt feelings or more excuses about why I didn't feel like having sex. Men equate sex with love, so no sex made Art feel distant and rejected. Not a great way to keep a marriage together, and the conflict was palpable.

> *Men equate sex with love, so no sex made Art feel distant and rejected.*

"Maybe you should talk to your doctor," Art suggested. "Maybe you're closer to menopause than you think and need some hormone therapy or something."

This was his response to one of those early morning passive-aggressive moments when I pretended to be asleep, so I wouldn't have to deal with sex. It didn't work. Art was rebuffed and not a happy man. I stared into the bathroom mirror, upset that I still had a little pooch.

"I've already been to the doctor, and she says it's probably just stress and the adrenal fatigue that's making me gain weight. I feel like a potato."

"You're still sexy to me, baby. You're sexy even in a potato sack," Art lovingly replied.

I sat on the side of the tub and started to sob. "I hate feeling like this."

Art held me close in a big bear hug and let me cry.

"I love you, baby, and I think you're very sexy. You can't expect to look like a teenager at fifty years old. You're too hard on yourself. Most women your age would kill to look like you."

He was right. Why was I beating myself up? I may not look like Christy Brinkley, but I wasn't a potato. I needed to make a plan to get my sexy back. I decided right then and there that I'd do the work to get back to my old self. Art still looked at me and told me he was the luckiest man in the world. Perhaps I only had to believe it. I decided that I wanted to be the woman that my husband adored.

After taking the adrenal supplements, changing my diet, and altering my exercise plan, I started feeling better and had less fatigue. I started weight training and doing abdominal exercises to lose the pooch. I stopped listening to all the negative self-talk and started to do more regular yoga to help with my body image. Positive affirmations and momentum helped me clear my mind of the impossible image I had of myself. I knew I would never look like my eighteen-year-old daughter, but I could be the best possible version of myself at fifty.

> *Positive affirmations and momentum helped me clear my mind of the impossible image I had of myself.*

I realized that being sexy was a mindset, not a body type. The only things in life I had complete control over every day were my attitude and effort. I decided to be sexy! So what if I had a few more curves? I went shopping for clothes that made me feel sexy and fit better. I even bought matching sexy underwear. Lace under my scrubs made me feel sexy, like I was doing something illegal. I got a new haircut and highlights. I got my nails done, got a facial, and changed up my makeup routine. New lipstick made me feel sexier.

Now on Friday nights, I would take a bubble bath, put on a lovely dress, perfume, makeup, and a pair of high heel shoes. I worked on feeling sexy to set the stage. I would even take a selfie of Art and me before we went out for dinner and post it on Instagram or Facebook. My social media following was always very complimentary, and that helped me start to believe my new positive mindset. I strutted into the restaurant with my head up high, feeling I had something to look at finally. We were actually a stunning couple when I got out of my sweatshirts and yoga pants.

The most important thing I did was being honest with Art. Instead of faking it or ignoring him, I told him if I wasn't up to sex or in the mood. He suggested that we start with a little cuddling, and then more often than not, it led to soft stroking. Somehow, sex started to look more appealing when I was lying in his arms.

When we were rehabbing my sleep problems, we got a new comfy bed and very soft sheets. I stopped wearing flannel pajamas and started sleeping naked or in a sexy nightgown again. I felt sexy when I slept naked. We worked on it together. We changed up our routines and communicated. We both made an effort. As with everything else, my sex drive started to come back as I began to recover from my adrenal fatigue. I still had some perimenopausal symptoms, but I could overcome them with some effort.

As with everything else, my sex drive started to come back as I began to recover from my adrenal fatigue.

I decided to love my body as it was and not compare it to its thirty-year-old self. As my body started to look better and feel better, I felt sexier. Art was always complimentary, and that helped as well. Positive talk between us was almost a daily affirmation. We set the stage with date nights and planned rendezvouses. There's nothing sexier than planning hotel sex in the middle of a Tuesday afternoon when you're usually at work. I highly recommend it!

8

I CAN'T THINK STRAIGHT

What was wrong with me? I was suffering from brain fatigue or some kind of brain fog. I was distracted, irritable, scattered, and couldn't think clearly. I'd wake up most days with a dull headache behind my eyes. It slowly went away when I drank a lot of water, but on some days, I felt like I was losing my mind. The headache came and went, but the ditzy blonde version of me stuck.

"Give me a minute, Sasha," I muttered as I slowly sipped my coffee.

"Mom," she repeated, "I need your help with this math problem. I forgot to do my homework, and the bus comes in a few minutes. Mom? Mom, are you listening to me?"

Taking a deep breath, I shuffled to the kitchen counter, trying to focus past my pounding headache.

"What do you have, baby?"

"Just algebra, but I don't get this one." Sasha shoved the piece of paper in my face, and I was met with $[-36x + 42x = 156]$.

"You want me to do math this early in the morning?" I asked with a soft chuckle.

In reality, it should have been easy for me. I mean, heck, I got an A in college calculus. I could do simple sixth-grade math.

Grasping the paper, I muttered, "Let me take a look while you pack up the rest of your stuff."

Typically, algebra was pretty simple for me, and I could do it in my head—but the brain fog, which was significantly worse in the morning, was crippling this morning. I couldn't sleep the night before, so I drank a little bit too much wine to turn off my brain. The pounding headache was starting to subside with my first cup of coffee, but the numbers on the page made no sense to me.

"Why don't you go see your math teacher when you get off the bus?" I suggested as she finished packing her backpack.

A stomping Sasha snatched the paper out of my hand and headed for the door. "Thanks, Mom, you're no help," she answered as she slammed the front door.

Another stellar Mom moment to add to my collection.

I felt helpless and defeated. I couldn't think straight anymore. Performing higher cognitive functions required focus. I would chalk it up to my sleeping problems, too much alcohol, and perimenopause, but these brain lapses didn't fit the profile. If it were only a hangover, my head would be clearer as the day progressed, and I wouldn't have persistent pain. If it was stress and fatigue, I should function better after sleeping most of the weekend.

I was starting to think I was losing my mind. Maybe I was starting down the road to early Alzheimer's or dementia. I was distracted and irritable most of the time. I was a bitch to everyone. I did stupid things like putting the milk in the pantry and the cereal in the refrigerator. I'd lost my car keys, my wallet, and a large check. Thank God, I cleaned my avalanche of a desk and found it. I even forgot to pick up Sasha from golf lessons. Maybe I had lost my mind.

I couldn't think straight anymore. Performing higher cognitive functions required focus. I would chalk it up to my sleeping problems, too much alcohol, and perimenopause, but these brain lapses didn't fit the profile.

I was at a loss. All I knew was that I had to fix this. My life, job, and family depended on it. Higher-level thinking was required to function as a physician and an entrepreneur.

So, I went back to Dr. Reed to see if I could find a solution.

"Tell me about your brain fog," she said.

"It's like I can't think anymore. I have a photographic memory, but I forget random things. I feel like I'm losing my mind. I can't focus," I explained. "Could this be early dementia? Or does every fifty-year-old woman go through this?"

"A certain amount of brain fog isn't uncommon during perimenopause," she said, "and it usually subsides after menopause. But your symptoms sound different than most. Is your sleeping getting any better with the progesterone?"

"A little bit, but some nights I can't turn off the noise in my head," I answered. "And I'm probably still drinking too much in an attempt to help me sleep," I confessed in almost a whisper.

"That's not helping," Dr. Reed replied. "I thought we worked through the nightly drinking. Are you still seeing the therapist?"

"Yes, and most of the time, I'm much better, but lately, I'm exhausted and can't think, so I find myself falling back into the old pattern," I answered honestly.

"If you get this sleep pattern fixed, I believe your brain function and thinking skills will get better. Let's run another spit test and see if your adrenals are getting any better. I also want to check your thyroid function because low thyroid can cause a foggy brain. Recovery from adrenal fatigue and chronic stress takes time." She closed my chart and started to fill out the lab slip.

"I get it," I answered with a deep sigh, "but I wish I could explain that to my staff and my kids. They all think I'm going crazy."

"It's probably time to have that chat with your partners about slowing down and even retiring. You need to take this seriously," Dr. Reed answered.

"I am, but it's hard to admit that I'm not ten feet tall and can't leap tall buildings in a single bound. I've managed a demanding life for years. Why can't I do it anymore?" I asked.

"Maybe you've burned the candle at both ends and have run out of wax, my friend. I don't have all the answers, but I know we can find a solution together. Everything still points to adrenal fatigue. You need to start accepting it and start making a plan to change your lifestyle—or you'll never feel better," Dr. Reed reprimanded as she left the room.

The door slammed. I got it. She was busy and was sick of repeating herself. And I was stubborn.

I couldn't be an effective leader if I was an irritable, forgetful bitch all the time. It was time to go back to the family therapist, Dr. Peters. Maybe she'd have some more concrete solutions for me.

"Tell me when you noticed the forgetfulness," Dr. Peters said. "Is it getting worse, or is it pretty much the same? Are you having problems with normal daily functions like getting out of bed and taking a shower? Or are you distracted and notice things like lost keys and forgotten appointments?"

I got comfortable in the soft, cushy chair. "Well, it gets worse as the week goes on, and no, I don't have problems with daily functions. I feel forgetful and scattered. Like I'm channeling my inner blonde." I laughed, trying to bring a little humor into all this crap.

"It's usually worse first thing in the morning, occasionally at the office when I'm stressed, and then later at night when I'm tired. My desk at the office looks like something blew up, and I usually feel way better when I'm organized. I'm irritable and scattered when I get home and feel overwhelmed trying to be everything for the girls after a long day. There doesn't seem to be any pattern to it that I can surmise."

"How are you doing with your alcohol control? Are you still drinking too much?" she asked.

"I'm getting it under control most days," I replied, slumping forward in the chair and looking at the floor. "Do you think I should go to a neurologist for a dementia screen? Or do I need to give up on trying to plan when I drink and go cold turkey into sobriety? Is that the answer? Do you think this is all from alcohol? If so, why isn't it getting any better? I rarely drink more than one or two glasses of wine and not even close to every day."

"We've had this discussion before, Marybeth," she firmly answered. "You have to decide if you can control your drinking. If you can't, and your log shows you can't, it's time to stop. And no, I don't think you need a neurologist, but I do think you have the perfect storm of stress, chaos, sleep disruption, too much alcohol, and way too much multitasking. You need to slow down and take these problems seriously. I know that's what your physician probably said as well."

"Sounds like the jury's in. I don't crave alcohol, and most days, I've been doing well with controlling my drinking or not having a drink at all, so I guess I'm not an alcoholic. I'm trying to do too much and fix everything all at the same time," I summarized, sitting up straighter in the chair.

"I agree with your assessment of your situation. Unless your labs come back with something new, I agree with Dr. Reed."

She got up from her chair and moved toward me, placing her hand on my shoulder. "Superwoman Syndrome needs to go. You can't keep up this charade much longer, and you shouldn't try."

It was time to drop the "S." This wasn't a defeat or a failure. I had to surrender in order to save me from myself.

I saw that all of my complaints were intertwined. I needed to get the sleep disorder under control. I needed to decrease my daily stress by cutting down my schedule. I needed to get back to a less stressful but more regular exercise program, and I needed to control my drinking and improve my hydration. Add a cleaner diet to that, and I should be perfect. Simple! *Not!* Old habits are hard to break.

It took some time and lots of daily changes, but I slowly began feeling more like myself. The brain fog began to clear after I made a plan and stuck to it. Here are the steps I took:

1. I slept at least eight hours every night.
2. I stopped trying to multitask.
3. I organized my desk and got rid of the vertical stacking method, which caused me to lose things.
4. I put my phone away when I was with patients or my girls. I was much less distracted and fully present with what was in front of me instead of continually getting updates or notifications.

5. I took off my Apple watch. It was a constant distraction. I used it only when running.

6. I decreased my social media interaction to twice a day and at specific times.

7. I only answered emails in the morning and before I left the office. My autoresponder prompted the sender to call if it was an emergency or if they needed an answer right away.

8. I talked with the other doctors in my practice and stopped taking overnight and weekend calls.

9. I turned my cell phone ringer off at eight o'clock every night. My family knew my home phone number if there was an emergency. Yes, I still had a home phone!

10. I decreased my clinic time to three days a week with a half-day on Friday for surgeries. This allowed me to eventually transition into retirement.

11. I asked the girls to help more around the house, and Caitlin even jumped in and did the grocery shopping since she had her driver's license.

12. I started reading before bed instead of watching TV—a real book, not an e-book.

13. I practiced crossword puzzles and sudoku to help my cognitive function.

14. I embraced short naps on my days off. These were also quite helpful in rejuvenating my brain. A twenty-minute power nap after lunch certainly made me more productive.

The change in routine improved my fatigue. My pseudo-dementia symptoms or brain fog started to lift. No more hangovers from alcohol and sleep deprivation. No more ditzy blonde! As my physical body was beginning to recover with sleep, diet, and exercise, my mental faculties returned. Once I took all my symptoms seriously and decided I didn't want to live in emotional pain and confusion anymore, I started to feel like myself again. I wanted to be free of Superwoman Syndrome.

9

THERE'S NEVER ENOUGH MONEY

Money has always been one of my primary emotional stress triggers. There never seemed to be enough, and no matter how much I made, we had an insatiable appetite for spending it.

I grew up in a small rural town where everyone was lower-middle class, blue collar, working class, and none of us had much. During the late seventies, the nearby union plants, where most dads worked if they weren't farming, seemed like they were always on strike. We knew what could be bought with food stamps and could agree on the quality of government cheese. At one point, my mother was working three jobs to keep us fed, housed, and clothed. I was oblivious and thought it was great that my mom worked the midnight shift at the donut shop since I got day-old donuts all the time!

Some of my earliest memories were of fights between my parents about money. My mother repeatedly told me how expensive it was to have three kids. Almost from birth, my mother told my sister and me to study hard, get good grades, and get a scholarship to college, so we would get out of that small town and be somebody. I think my mother always resented not being able to go to college and being stuck in our small hometown.

I never realized we were poor until I went to junior high and was thrust into a regional junior-senior high school with four neighboring towns. The differences between the haves and have nots were evident—like the hand-me-down clothes from my sister versus designer Izod shirts. Let the bullying and fashion-shaming begin. Junior high girls were mean!

My pathological relationship with money was due to my childhood programming, and there probably isn't enough therapy to undo it.

All kidding aside, I hated being one of the poor kids. I was determined to be successful and come back to my high school reunions and rub it in some of the mean girls' faces. I played by the rules, got good grades, went to college on a full scholarship, and even managed to get a medical school scholarship. I got out of that small town and learned along the way that money doesn't make you happy, but man, it can make you much more comfortable.

I was still in my first marriage in 2008, and there never seemed to be enough money. I had a busy, profitable practice and a growing family who appeared to have an unbelievable ability to spend every dollar I made. We had all the trappings of success: the big house, the Mercedes, the overseas vacations, and the expensive wardrobes. At the time, my husband's business wasn't doing well. He always seemed to need a little extra help to pay his bills.

"Jim, this is ridiculous," I lamented as I walked into the kitchen and saw the beach towels surrounding the base of the dishwasher. "We have to replace the dishwasher. It's leaking even worse now."

. . . money doesn't make you happy, but man, it can make you much more comfortable.

There was a puddle seeping onto the tile floor, even with four beach towels packed around it.

"It still works, and it doesn't leak that much," he replied over his shoulder as he headed for the garage.

"We need to talk about this!" I shouted at the back of his head. "Wait a minute, where are you going?"

"I need to meet a guy at the soccer center. The main freezer in the restaurant broke again!" he yelled from the garage.

"I'm going to Home Depot to order a new dishwasher!" I yelled back.

Jim turned around slowly and walked back into the kitchen, a concerned look on his face. He leaned against the granite island that housed the leaking mass.

"Honey, we can't afford a new dishwasher until things get better at the center. You're going to have to be patient."

Something exploded in my head at that point. I wouldn't have been surprised if I had an aneurysm.

"What?" I screamed. "I made high six figures last year, and we can't afford a fucking dishwasher? We need to figure this shit out! I can't work any more than I am, and you're making nothing. Your company is a hobby, not a job! I think it's time to sell the soccer center."

He took one look at my red face, turned on his heel, and headed out to his truck.

"We can talk when you calm down," he called back over his shoulder. "The dishwasher isn't a big deal. Make the girls wash the dishes."

And then he was gone. He left me sobbing on the tile floor, staring at the puddle. What the fuck? I'd had enough. I was working so hard to glean every dollar from my practice, and he was siphoning everything he could from the family coffers, so he didn't have to admit his business was failing.

I wish I could say this was our first fight about money. Jim's attitude was that we should spend what we had and then some. It was always *our* money, even when he wasn't making any. He liked having the big house and all the trappings of success. He was proud of his family. Admittedly, I was also guilty of trying to keep up with the Joneses. I liked it when people acknowledged how successful I was. I felt that because I worked so hard, I deserved to have nice things, even if we struggled with a little debt. Not being able to buy a new dishwasher was a wake-up call. That was a conversation that happened in my parents' house, not mine!

When we divorced in 2009, I thought my money issues were over. But they were only beginning. Jim got the house in Florida, the soccer center, a little acreage we had purchased, and his 1966 Corvette and truck. I got the house, the kids, my medical practice, and my SUV. I paid a bunch of credit card debt for the soccer center and felt like we had an agreement that worked.

After filing my taxes in 2010, I had quite a bit of money left over in my tax account and asked my accountant what I forgot to pay.

He said, "No, Marybeth, that's probably about as much money as your husband was regularly siphoning. Go buy something fun with it."

So, I did. I bought a Mercedes CLK convertible that I didn't need, but it was a cherry red "fuck you" car.

Life was humming along, and I was making great strides in repairing my finances when in early 2011, I received a certified letter from Bank of America. Curious, since I didn't bank there anymore. I opened it immediately and found a demand letter for $1.1 million, payable in thirty days. What? Stunned, I slid down the wall of the kitchen and sat on the floor. Yep, I was on the damn tile floor again. There had to be some mistake. I immediately called my lawyer.

"Did you sign a personal guarantee on the soccer center loan when you and Jim purchased it?" she asked me.

"I have no idea. I signed a lot of stuff since we used my credit to qualify for the SBA loan." There was a growing sense of dread in my stomach.

"You probably did. The banks don't have to follow the family court decree if you signed a personal guarantee."

"Fuck. What am I going to do now? I don't have $1.1 million in liquid assets. Hell, I don't think I have that kind of money period."

"You probably don't need to come up with all of it right away. The bank will play 'let's make a deal,'" she explained.

I was stunned and felt like vomiting or shooting Jim. How could he do this to the girls and me? I was taking care of the kids and not asking him for anything. I guess that wasn't enough.

The next morning, I called the bank, and it turned out that I had signed a personal guarantee for the SBA loan. Jim hadn't made any payments in over six months. I started to scramble. My divorce lawyer referred me to a commercial business lawyer who took care of this kind of issue. In a few weeks, we mortgaged my house, paid the bank enough for them to let me resume payments on the loan, evicted my ex-husband from the center, and found another soccer group to rent it out. The one thing I didn't do was shoot Jim. Most days, I still wanted to, but he was the girls' dad, so I let him live. I had put a tourniquet on the checkbook and avoided bankruptcy. Jim wasn't so lucky, and I wasn't empathetic.

I knew from past experience that money didn't buy happiness, but it certainly made me more secure and comfortable. There is stress in not having enough money, and this kind of stress contributed to my adrenal fatigue. It took me almost ten years to sell the soccer center, and many of my close friends heard a lot of cussing, crying, and screaming about that money pit. I vowed never to be that stupid about money again and never sign anything ever again without asking lots of questions.

> *There is stress in not having enough money, and this kind of stress contributed to my adrenal fatigue.*

I sold my big house and downsized to a smaller, more energy-efficient home. I gave up the extra bedrooms and five-car garage I didn't need anyway. I sold my convertible, turned in the SUV I'd been leasing, and bought a new SUV with cash. I paid off my mortgage and vowed to get entirely out of debt as soon as possible. All the extra money I had went to pay the debt. I achieved my debt-free milestone and then started saving half my income in a brokerage account. I fully funded the kids' college 529 plans, and my accountant told me I could retire whenever I wanted. I had systematically eliminated the majority of my money stressors. Having no debt and a nice nest egg was liberating. It felt amazing.

Before I remarried, one of the first discussions Art and I had about blending our lives was money. One of the most endearing things Art ever said to me was, "Honey, I want you to understand my feelings about debt. There is no good debt. Debt and different attitudes toward money were part of the demise of my first marriage. I want to make sure we're on the same page, or this isn't going to work."

Before the wedding, I rewrote my will and put all of my money in a trust for the girls. I wanted them to be secure no matter what happened.

In the years following the wedding, Art and I had many more discussions about money. We both reinforced why staying out of debt was so crucial to both of us. It was refreshing to be married to someone who had the same attitude toward money, although not quite as pathological. I still probably have an unhealthy relationship with money, but it no longer has the power it once had. I've learned that money can only stress you out if you let it.

Simple changes in your behavior can take power away from money.

1. Spend what you have. Sounds simple, but most Americans spend way more than they make.
2. Realize there is no good debt. There is fantastic security in not having any debt.
3. Keeping up with the Joneses is a fallacy. They're probably drowning in debt. According to Experian's 2019 Consumer Debt Study, the total consumer debt in the US was $14.1 trillion, with Americans carrying an average personal debt of $90,460!
4. Save as much as you comfortably can. Start with small amounts and increase as your earning ability increases. You could even get a little side gig to fund your savings. I used to lecture quite a bit for pharmaceutical

companies and banked all of the speaking fees. The law of compounding interest is very liberating in the long run, and you probably don't need that seven-dollar Starbucks coffee.

5. Diversify your investments. I have commercial real estate, mutual funds, stocks, bonds, and a little cash. It's incredible when one goes down, the rest go up, and vice versa. It's a game. Don't try to time the market; even the big boys can't do that.

6. Every time you want to buy something or spend a large amount of money, ask yourself, "Do I need this? Or do I just want it?" It's okay to splurge from time to time, as long as you aren't going into debt for it and are sticking to a systematic savings plan.

Money and I have agreed to a truce. Money doesn't have the power to make me crazy because I won't let it.

10

I'M SPIRITUALLY EMPTY

"When was the last time you took your kids to church?" my mother asked. "You know they need it, especially with all this turmoil in your house."

"Mom, they hate going, and I'm sick of fighting with them," I patiently answered. "I'm not going to force them to go like we had to when we were kids."

My mother sighed. "They need to have a close relationship with God to have any chance to be successful in this brazen world. Aren't you worried about their souls?"

"I'm so tired I'd rather sleep in on a Sunday, and I don't think God is intervening in our daily lives." Who had time for a God who let the whole world go mad?

Grief can make you question if there is some higher being orchestrating this puppet show. When my son was stillborn, I kept telling myself that God must be trying to prepare me for some purpose after the initial excruciating pain.

Pastor Nancy, who sat with me as I cried and lamented in the hospital, gave me some philosophical words to ponder.

"Marybeth, I know this loss is very hard, but I want you to realize that God sees the world from a different view. I've always felt that he sees a beautiful tapestry where all we can see is its underside, with all the knots and cut-off pieces. I truly believe that only when we are with the Lord can we fully appreciate his plan for the world." She hugged me and left me after praying for my healing.

After she left the sterile, cold hospital room, I thought, *God, why me? I'm healthy and did everything right during this pregnancy. I don't understand.* I think he planned to test my faith with a roller coaster ride until I finally reached to him for comfort.

God and I have always had a tumultuous relationship. I felt spiritually empty and didn't think there was some supreme being with whom I needed to have a relationship. I was wrong, and God has a way of teaching us that we need him. Amid my soccer center debacle, my real estate lawyer shared his faith and asked if he could pray for my situation. Coming from this seasoned junkyard dog of an attorney, I was stunned. I told him it couldn't hurt! The bank accepted our offer to pay the arrears and assume the loan the next day. Maybe prayers were answered, or this was only a coincidence. I wasn't convinced.

Twenty-four hours later, another God moment happened. I was thirty-five thousand dollars short on the bank payment after mortgaging my home and was trying to figure out how to scrape it up when my phone rang. It was the Mercedes salesman. I'm not sure why I even answered. I wasn't in any shape to buy a new car.

"Dr. Crane?"

"Yes, John. How are you?"

"I'm doing well but calling to ask you a silly question."

"What's up?" I replied, wondering where this was going.

"Do you still have that red CLK convertible?"

"Yes, why?"

"I have a lady who hates the new body style and is looking for the old one. Any thoughts of selling it? I can get you a new E Class convertible for a good price."

"No, John, I hadn't thought about it. I don't drive it that much. I pretty much drive my SUV with all the kids' activities, and I've got a lot going on right now, so a new car is probably not in the budget."

John paused and then asked, "How many miles do you have on it?"

"Let me check. Not a ton, probably eleven thousand or so."

"How about I buy it from you since you don't drive it much? I know it was an impulse buy," John replied. "I can give you thirty-five thousand and have you a check in forty-eight hours."

Stunned, I almost ended up on the kitchen floor again. "I think that's a great idea."

"Great," John replied. "I'll get the paperwork together and stop by your house to pick it up and give you the check."

Hanging up the phone, I fell on the couch and took a deep breath.

"Lord," I prayed, "Thank you, and please forgive me for my unfaithfulness. I don't deserve your mercy, but I'm grateful for your intercession." That God moment changed my heart for a while.

I had been spiritually empty and started believing religion was an opiate for the masses. I didn't think I needed it. Church was boring, and I often fell asleep during the sermon. My kids hated it after about eight years old. It was even more boring for them. My fatigue made it even easier to sleep in and let them as well. I didn't think God cared.

His mercy made me seek Him more, but it was several years before I pulled my head and heart out of my butt and got serious about seeking to find meaning in my relationship with God. He kept nudging me closer to Him with various God moments. Still, it wasn't until I reached rock

I had been spiritually empty and started believing religion was an opiate for the masses. I didn't think I needed it.

bottom and sought a respite from my unrelenting fatigue that I truly felt led to having a more personal relationship with my Lord and Savior Jesus Christ.

A strict Seventh Day Baptist Church upbringing meant going to church for hours every Saturday and never going out on Friday night after sundown because it was the Sabbath. Too many rules came with the church. My parents were an integral part of the SDB community, and our church family was close. Most of the teenagers felt the same way that I did. Potluck dinners were fantastic, but going to church was something you had to do so you didn't piss off your parents. My need for church stayed in my small hometown when I fled and ran away to college. I felt no need for God out in the big, bad world. That was a thing for my uneducated parents. I was wrong.

After Elise died In 2016, I found myself questioning my beliefs and even started to wonder whether or not there was a God.

In my car, I screamed, "Lord, where are you? How can you explain this to me? What purpose is served by the drowning death of an amazing thirteen-year-old?"

He never answered me, or I wasn't open to hearing him. I felt so alone and empty.

We were all devastated. After planning a funeral and propping up the family, none of us felt like we understood what kind of God could have taken this exceptional child. The priest seemed more interested in what type of donation we would give the church for the funeral mass than helping us deal with our grief.

Death often breeds anger. Anger and bitterness ate at my soul and made me feel emptier, hollow. I felt alone in my thoughts. About a year after Elise's death, I found myself yearning for meaning. I was so tired of being empty and sad. How could I help Lori deal with her grief if I felt so dreadful? In my darkest hour, the Lord opened a window for me when the door of my soul seemed firmly locked.

In the still of my early morning meditation, I clearly heard, "Marybeth, you can't help Lori heal if you don't start taking care of yourself."

Lord, is that you? I cried out in my mind to the rising sun.

"I've always been here. How many times have I reached out to you, and yet you still reject me? When will you realize that I'm in control, and you should leave the responsibility of fixing everyone and everything to me?"

He made me long for his peace. The conversation was as clear as day.

My physician encouraged me to start a meditation practice in the early morning to mitigate my stress, but what I heard in the quiet, still moments were all these whispers in my brain. It was like God was talking directly to me about what was going on in my life. I started to listen. Meditation turned into quiet prayer time, and I felt a two-way communication with the Lord.

I started a Bible study on grief. We started going back to church, but a completely different one. I sought one out that energized kids and teens. At Gateway Church, we found a home. I started going to weeknight Bible study for single moms, which made me realize I was blessed. So many of the women were having trouble supporting themselves and their kids. The motivational pastors were all about forgiving yourself and your ex. That took a while, but I first forgave myself for my own indiscretions, then forgave Jim for all the pain he inflicted on me. A heavy weight lifted, and I realized that all the anger was part of my stress and fatigue as well.

Gateway Church was instrumental in my spiritual recovery. Pastor Robert's sermon on the power of prayer hit home.

He stated, "Prayer is a two-way conversation with God. Cast your burdens at the feet of Jesus!" He then quoted Philippians 4:6-7: "Be anxious for nothing, but in everything by prayer and supplication, with thanksgiving, let your requests be made known to God; and the peace of God, which surpasses all understanding, will guard your hearts and minds through Christ Jesus." (NKJV)

God heard my daily prayers. The voice I heard in the early morning was God. I felt it in my soul. Every day, I felt a little better. A little lighter. The Lord was changing my life; I had to stop being stubborn and give Him the reins.

A pivotal change happened. I started a daily gratitude journal and then decided to spread positivity with daily affirmational posts on my Facebook page. The affirmations lifted my mood, and my physical fatigue improved when my mental outlook was more positive. I stopped listening to the negative self-talk and started listening to the calming whispers in the early morning. God is good, and He's got this! There's no other way we can survive in this world! The enemy is continually trying to turn you away from God. No eternal fatigue is stronger than my God!

I only have to remember my mantra, Matthew 7:7, "Ask, and it shall be given you; seek, and ye shall find; knock, and it shall be opened unto you." (KJV)

I prayed when I felt the urge to shoulder all the responsibility of fixing Lori's world: "Lord, I know I don't deserve your mercy and grace, but please take this burden from my heart."

"I already have, my child. Let me. Surrender it to me." I heard His voice as clear as day.

I made prayer a priority. Miraculously, I felt lighter each day. I felt His peace. I knew He was listening and would guide my recovery. And I knew He had Lori in his arms and would work on helping her find her way back to Him. It wasn't my responsibility to fix her, only to love her.

I know that I will never be able to completely understand the roller coaster ride that I've been living in this life, but when I'm standing next to my Lord, I know I will be okay. I firmly believe it. I want this calming peace for all of us. Can I get an Amen?

11

I'M SO OVERWHELMED

When Art and I had only been married a few months, Caitlin made homemade chocolate chip cookies—her favorite food in the universe. Not wanting to share them, she hid them at the top of one of the kitchen cupboards. Later that day, Art found them, and the two had words about sharing. Art told Caitlin that we were a family and should share everything. That included cookies. Caitlin told him that she made them, so she didn't have to share. Art proceeded to eat one and said that even though she'd made them, he bought the groceries, so they were for everyone. She stomped off to her room in typical teenage fashion. Of course, that wasn't the end of it.

The next evening, I came rushing home from work on a wing and a prayer to take Caitlin to CrossFit and found her sobbing uncontrollably on the kitchen floor.

"Mom," Caitlin whimpered, "Art took my cookies and won't tell me where they are."

Exasperated, I replied, "What are you talking about? Are we still arguing about cookies?"

"Yes, and he is a total jerk off!"

Art and Caitlin had had a very heated text exchange, and she'd told him how much of a jerk he was. He was trying to make a point, and she was acting like he'd killed her puppy. They were both being ridiculous. I was exhausted and scooped her up, picked up her carpool buddy, and took them to CrossFit.

I went home to help Sasha with her homework and forgot all about the cookies. A little more than an hour later, a sweaty Caitlin walked into the house with a couple dozen cookies from the local bakery. The other carpool mom had heard the cookie story and thought it was silly, so she picked up cookies on the way home. I snapped a picture of us all eating cookies and sent it to Art with the caption that now we had plenty of cookies to share.

Bad idea. He was even more pissed.

I got a text that stated, *If you don't want me to try to parent your children, then maybe I shouldn't care at all.*

Oops! I'd poked the bear. I poured a glass of wine, ate a cookie, and shooed everyone off to bed. When Art got home later that night, I was asleep. The next day, he again reminded me that he could either help raise my children or stay out of it, but he wasn't going to do it halfway.

Over the next few weeks, Caitlin was still adamant that she'd done nothing wrong and Art was a jerk. She repeated that to him and added that he wasn't her father, so she didn't need to listen to him. The two of them barely spoke, and when they did, it was through snippy, sarcastic comments.

This went on for over a month, with me playing referee. Life was hectic enough without this chaos. Suddenly, the sweet, loving man I married had no interest in being a parent to my children and no interest in their achievements. He didn't even want to go to Caitlin's track meets because he was so pissed at her behavior.

One evening, I was sitting in the living room, falling asleep on my incredibly comfortable couch with my feet up on the ottoman. I was enjoying a nice glass of Cabernet after a long day. Art had come home, poured himself a glass of wine, and sat on the couch to watch a movie with me. Caitlin wandered into the living room, and Art made a sarcastic remark to Caitlin about how even I shared my wine.

I'd had it. I threw my wine glass at the wall and fell into a sobbing heap on the ottoman. The shattered glass was at Caitlin's feet, and she stood still as a statue. She had that look in her eyes like, *What just happened?*

"I can't take this anymore!" I cried. "If you two don't stop fighting, I'm going to lose it."

Well, I guess I already did.

They both stared at me with disbelief.

"The whole world is a conspiracy against me!" I cried. "It's bad enough that I have to play referee every day at the office. I can't take this anymore."

I got up and rushed to my bedroom. I was physically and emotionally exhausted. I felt like a complete failure as a mother and wife.

Caitlin ran to her room in typical teenage fashion while Art cleaned up the shards of glass.

Once he cleaned up the broken glass, Art went upstairs and apologized to Caitlin for letting this go so far, then told her, "Go downstairs and see what our stubbornness has done to your mother."

I was under my covers, still sobbing.

"Mom, I love you, and I'm sorry we upset you," Caitlin whispered.

"It's okay, baby," I whimpered back. "I've just had a bad day." *Or month*, I thought to myself.

The cookie saga was over. Maybe I should've thrown something sooner.

Family dynamics will always default to stupid and stubborn unless you intervene. Men are just big kids, and kids are just that—kids. Conflict is inevitable, and avoidance makes it fester until someone explodes—or throws a wine glass. Their behavior wasn't my responsibility, but somehow, I owned it. I was overwhelmed at the office and at home. I felt like a failure everywhere.

It felt like I was watching a soap opera of someone

I was overwhelmed at the office and at home. I felt like a failure everywhere.

else's life. I mostly played by the rules. I worked hard, went to school, got married, built the business, had kids along the way, and woke up exhausted all the time. I felt like I was doing a shitty job at just about everything. When did things get so out of control? What happened?

The cookie caper is a great example. I should've stopped it initially, but I was too tired to nip it in the bud until it spiraled out of control.

I knew that I needed to communicate better with my family. We needed to talk about how I was feeling. Not long after the cookie caper, we had a family meeting.

"Gang," I said, sitting on the couch surrounded by my tribe, "We have to discuss how I'm feeling. I'm not proud of chucking a wine glass a few weeks ago, but it certainly got your attention."

"You scared the shit out of me," Caitlin said sheepishly. "I hadn't seen you act like that since I cut my bangs when I was six years old. You were so pissed I thought your head was going to explode."

"Yes, Caitlin, I was angry, and I should've knocked both of your heads together from the beginning. The situation spiraled out of control so fast," I said.

"Why am I here?" my sweet Sasha asked. "I had nothing to do with the stolen cookies."

"You're here because Mommy wants to talk with all of you."

"Okay. About what?" Sasha asked.

"About some changes that we need to make around here," I answered.

"What kind of changes?" Caitlin asked.

"I think your mother needs you girls to help a little more around the house," Art interjected.

"Not just the girls. I need your help too," I said. "It'll take a group effort and better communication to distribute the housework, so I can stop feeling so overwhelmed."

"What do you want me to do?" asked Sasha.

"Not be such a brat! And do your homework without Mom," interjected Caitlin.

"Stop it, you two," I retorted, getting up from the couch and pacing around the living room.

"Sasha, you can start walking the dog when you get home from school. I walk him every morning at five-thirty. The least you can do is take him for his afternoon walk."

"But, Mom, I have a ton of homework," Sasha whined.

"So do I," I replied, pointing to my briefcase and computer bag. "It will take you fifteen minutes and take one chore off my plate. You wanted a dog, so perhaps you should help with his care."

"Okay," she said. "I guess I can start doing that. But even when it's raining?"

"Yes, even when it's raining," I chuckled.

Turning to back to Caitlin, I said, "And I need you two to pick up your shit downstairs and stop having the house look like a tornado went through it. And you're old enough to do your own laundry. I'd like you to add to the grocery list when you eat the last of something, and, Caitlin, I want you to start doing the grocery shopping. You have free time Thursday afternoons, and it would prevent me from having to fight the crowds on Saturday mornings."

"What about me?" Art asked. "What do you want me to do?"

"Could you wash the dishes when I cook and maybe even cook once in a while? While you're at it, you could pick up your stuff too," I said.

"I definitely can be your chief dishwasher and perhaps your once-a-week pizza man. And yes, I will be more mindful of dropping my stuff everywhere," Art answered.

"I can cook," Sasha added.

"I think that would give Mom more stress," Caitlin said. "You'd probably burn down the house."

"No, I wouldn't, you jerk," Sasha snapped.

"Perhaps you can help, Sasha. You could be my prep cook and learn along the way," I suggested. "Honestly, girls, it's more the chaos of trying to keep up with your stuff that's strewn all over the house. I could have a yard sale just from stuff on the dining room table that we never use.

"I know I've been very cranky lately. If you help decrease my daily stress, hopefully, I'll start getting back to my normal sweet self."

"Sweet?" Caitlin chuckled.

"When have I not been sweet Mom?"

"Keep telling yourself that," Caitlin answered. "You've always been mean Mom!"

"That, my daughter, is completely not true," I laughed. "Family meeting adjourned."

That was great! A simple but effective family meeting where I explained my needs, asked for simple help, and distributed responsibilities. I wasn't selfish; I was exercising self-care.

As part of Superwoman Syndrome, I had taken on all the household responsibilities without teaching the family to help. Learned helplessness was what I'd taught my children and my husband. I even took on the guilt and responsibility for their poor behaviors, like with the cookie caper. Life in our house was about to change.

As part of Superwoman Syndrome, I had taken on all the household responsibilities without teaching the family to help.

With Superwoman Syndrome, you expect to be the perfect wife, the perfect mother, and a workaholic at the same time. I'm not sure how that works in anyone's reality, but it didn't work in mine. I think a lot of us fake it. We hold on by our fingernails. Try not to show the chinks in our armor. The mask of perfection cannot fall off. We pretend to live our Facebook life.

Next, I had a meeting with the other doctors about workload distribution. We decided that if someone at the office could do 75 percent of the job as well as I could, then it needed to be delegated. I had to slow down my clinical and administrative responsibilities. In the end, I felt like I could never make a dent on my to-do list. So, it was time to chuck the to-do list.

While I thought I was the only one who was struggling to keep it together, over a drink with a friend, I realized this wasn't true.

"Amanda, how do you keep it all together?" I asked as I took another sip of wine, looking around her immaculate home.

"What do you mean?"

"You're a lawyer, mother of two great kids, you seem to actually like your husband, you're fit and trim, and your house looks perfect. What's your secret?"

"I'm faking it," she answered, laughing. "My kids are little shits. Chloe is about to fail eighth-grade math, and Sam is a little hormonal bitch most of the time. I barely talk to my husband when he's home. He travels all the time. I barely eat anything to keep the weight off. My kids eat macaroni and cheese and hot dogs because I'm too tired to cook. And the cleaning lady was here this morning. Why do you think I invited you over today?"

"So, you're having trouble balancing everything too?" I asked in disbelief. She always seemed to have an organized home and the perfect world.

"Sister, ask any woman in the neighborhood who has a job, let alone is a professional. They'll tell you the same thing: we're all faking it. Welcome to the façade of the perfect little affluent family. I would even bet that most of the women, if they were honest, are going pretty insane."

"Wow, I'm stunned. Perhaps it would help if we talked about what was going on in our lives instead of fostering the Facebook reality we show to everyone. We should start a little group therapy for the neighborhood women."

"The problem is that no one wants to be judged by what they perceive are failures. None of us are perfect, but most of us won't admit it and keep trying," Amanda said. "We're our own worst enemies."

The only escape from this trap is to admit that life isn't perfect, accept it, then internalize it.

Not long after my wine-sipping session with Amanda, I started a working moms group. I invited the women I knew who were probably also struggling. I broke the ice by telling my story, and then they opened up. I thought my household was a disaster, but each of us had a similar story to tell about trying to do everything and be everything for everybody. Superwoman Syndrome was an epidemic.

Superwoman Syndrome was an epidemic.

"Marybeth, I can't believe the craziness that's gone on in your life," Sandy said as she poured another glass of wine. We were sitting in my backyard enjoying the sunset with five other neighborhood ladies. The moms group was a monthly affair and helped all of us cope.

"I think I would've killed your ex by now," Amy added.

"I had no idea, and I live right next door, and Tara rides the bus with Sasha," Meredith interjected. "But really, at least you have the income to shoulder it all. If my ex stopped paying me, I'd have to move. Can't keep this train running on my teacher's salary."

"I think that's part of the problem," I said. "Jim knew I could do it all, so he let me. A little help would have been nice."

"Well, when they help, they usually make you pay for it in other ways. When did life get so hard? And men get so stupid?" Meredith asked.

"I think it's always been this way, but our mothers hid it from us pretty well," Amy answered with a chuckle. "I think they were afraid that if they told us the truth, they wouldn't ever have any grandkids!"

"A little heads-up would've been helpful," I said wryly.

"We wouldn't have listened anyway. Think about how well our kids listen to us," Meredith said, laughing.

We laughed and cried over the train wreck that was most of our lives, but we also talked each other off the ledge—and we started to let the façade crack and peel. We needed a safe space to be real. We all needed a sisterhood to lean on. Communicating with other women who suffered from Superwoman Syndrome was enlightening and empowering. It made me feel less alone.

12

I'M SUCH A PERFECTIONIST

"Do you know how hard it is to be your daughter?" Alex screamed at me. "You think I should be perfect at everything, just like you!"

"Honey, calm down. I'm not telling you to be perfect. And I'm certainly not perfect. I'm merely suggesting that perhaps you should try a little harder," I calmly replied, then sat on the couch, trying to keep my cool. Seventh grade had been hard on Alex, and her grades had suffered.

"This test is not your best work. Did you study?" I asked.

"Of course, I studied, but when will you get it? I'm more like Dad than you, and school is stupid!" she lamented as she stomped away to her room. "And the teacher is an idiot!" she shouted over her shoulder.

She returned quickly with a backpack on her shoulder and barked, "I called Grandpa. I'm heading over there, so I can be with people who appreciate me for me. Face it, Mom, I'll never be that perfect child you want me to be. At least Dad and Grandma let me be me!"

A horn beeped outside, and she was gone. Her paternal grandparents, who lived only a mile away, were her oasis in the desert of our relationship.

Alex and I barely spoke anymore. She blamed me for the divorce and didn't even listen to my point of view. Maybe I did push her too hard, but I was successful because I was so driven. Was it wrong to hope she would be successful in life as well?

Her father let her slide through life as he had. School wasn't important to him. He never finished college. He wasn't shouldering any of the girls' financial burdens and kept making excuses for not being able to help. The only thing he did on a regular basis to be their father was show up at all their school functions and sporting events. Otherwise, the girls went to his parents' house on Friday nights and the occasional full weekend when I was out of town. Sometimes, he was also there because that's where he lived at the time, and sometimes, he was out of town. Grandma and Grandpa were always reliable.

I was afraid that if Alex followed her father's example, her life wouldn't be the one of her dreams. I wanted more for her. I wanted her to have the life choices only available with higher education. I still loved her and wanted the best life for her, no matter the conflict.

After the door slammed, I lay down on the couch and started to sob. I felt helpless. Caitlin had run down the hall to her room and slammed her door to get out of the fray. Sasha, from her spot on the living room floor, watched the madness, appearing to be oblivious of what was going on. Ignorance was bliss, and she seemed to be a happy kid who played with her toys. At five, she most likely understood way more than she was showing but didn't react to the sideshow.

It was time to call Dr. Peters. I needed to talk to someone, and she always answered my calls, even on the weekends.

Dr. Peters answered on the second ring.

"Sorry to bother you. It's Alex again. She left to go to her grandparents for the third time this week. I'm afraid one of these days she won't come back," I lamented.

In her soft, calming voice, Dr. Peters counseled, "Marybeth, take a deep breath. She's a thirteen-year-old girl, and her world is in turmoil. She feels that you are the enemy."

"Why do I have to be the enemy when I'm the only one holding this household together? Her dad doesn't even help," I asked, trying to keep from crying and upsetting Sasha. I tried to calm down and look at least outwardly normal.

"I suck at this and everything else lately. I can't think straight, and Alex wants to fight all the time."

"How are the other girls?" asked Dr. Peters.

"Caitlin is hiding in her room, so she doesn't have to be around the screaming. Sasha's only five, so she's either oblivious or has decided not to get involved. She's happily playing. What am I doing wrong?" I asked as I got off the couch and started toward my bedroom. "I'm working my ass off so they have everything they need and want. I'm exhausted, and I feel like a big, hot mess."

"Perhaps you should relax and not be so judgmental of Alex and yourself," Dr. Peters suggested. "She's a teenage girl, which means she's a hormonal disaster on top of the turmoil in your lives. Cut her some slack. She feels pulled back and forth between you and Jim. She doesn't have to take sides, but she hasn't realized that. One day she will, but until then, one of you has to be the bad guy, and today it's you. It's okay not to be perfect all the time. While you're at it, give yourself a break too. Trying to be Superwoman is wearing on you."

Perhaps she was right. I hated my mother as a teenager because she pushed me so hard. I had to study hard and get good grades. She even threatened to keep me from running cross country because it took me away from my studies.

I took some deep, cleansing breaths. I thanked Dr. Peters for her advice and found Caitlin huddled in her closet. In the back reaches of the dark closet, far away from the chaos. This turmoil wasn't healthy for any of us, especially her.

"Caitlin, it's okay. You can come out. Don't make me crawl back there and get you," I said as I opened the closet door wider and turned on the light.

"Is she gone?" Caitlin asked in a whisper. "I hate it when you fight."

"I know, baby. I try not to fight with Alex, but she keeps pushing my buttons," I replied as she came out of the closet and into my open arms.

I hugged her close and slumped to the floor. I cradled her like she was five, not eleven. We sat for a minute, and I rocked her in my arms, smoothing out her blonde hair.

"Are you okay?" I asked.

"I'm okay. Just don't stop holding me. You know Alex wants to go live with Grandma? She thinks that will fix everything. She told me I should demand to come with her, too, Mommy, but I don't want to. I don't want to leave you alone. I love you, Mommy. Don't worry, I won't leave you." Caitlin hugged me closer as she spoke these precious words.

At least Caitlin and Sasha needed and loved me. I could only pray that one day, Alex would see the light.

"Come on, Caitlin," I said as I wiped the tears from her face, "Let's go find Sasha and make some dinner. I'm hungry, and I bet you are too."

"Can we have ice cream?" Caitlin asked as she stood up and headed for the kitchen.

"Sure, why not?" Why not have ice cream for dinner? It's been that kind of day.

We found Sasha still playing with her dolls in the living room. Bless that child. A hurricane went through the living room with all kinds of yelling and slamming doors, but she appeared to be happy as a little clam.

I've always been a perfectionist. I had to be the best at everything I did, or I was disappointed in myself. I could almost hear my mother in my head chanting, "You can do better than that. Is this your best effort? Second is not good enough."

I was my biggest critic. Self-love and self-compassion were not words in my vocabulary. Good enough was never good enough; I had to be the best. I'm not sure if I was born that way or programmed by my mother. Either way, perfection was at the core of my personality.

> *I could almost hear my mother in my head chanting, "You can do better than that. Is this your best effort? Second is not good enough."*

Several weeks after Alex stormed out of the house, I got a certified letter from my ex. He wanted custody of Alex and felt it was the best thing for everyone. In the state of Texas, a twelve-year-old child can choose who they wanted to live with, even if that parent didn't have an income and still lived with his parents three years after the divorce. Dr. Peters agreed that Alex should spend at least the summer with her grandparents and her father. This would allow

Caitlin and Sasha a little more normalcy, and it might decrease my stress. She felt that, over time, Alex would come to realize the divorce wasn't all one-sided. She told me to let her go and that she would come back eventually.

That was in 2011. Jim won the custody battle for Alex in the Fall of 2011, after she spent the summer with him at her paternal grandparents. The court let her choose. Fast forward to 2015. Alex spent all of her high school years at her grandparents' house. We barely spoke unless she needed something, usually money or a signature. She rarely came over to the house and never slept in the room I prepared for her in our new home. I tried to bridge the gap, but I was banging my head against a stone wall.

Caitlin and Sasha were much better without her volatility in the house. Caitlin and I got close. She was a sophomore in high school by this point and had a different perspective. She was running cross country and loved to share her workouts with me. I was proud of her and cherished our relationship but still wished I could reach Alex.

"Mom, Alex is never going to believe Dad is wrong about anything. You might as well accept it," Caitlin advised.

"I can't, Caitlin. Doesn't she see that I'm the one holding all this together?" I answered. My argument hadn't changed.

"She doesn't believe it, even if I throw it in her face, Mom. I often hate being around her because she always wants to argue and defend Dad. She loves tearing you apart. She's moving to Florida in the fall to go to college, and I'm happy. I hate how she makes you so upset."

I hated hearing these words from Caitlin. I had always envisioned my girls as a tribe that loved and supported each other as they aged. I'm not sure why, since my sister and I are not close. She would take a bullet for me, and I for her, but we barely talk more than at the obligatory holidays or when we have exciting or tragic news. We are different people with completely divergent ideals.

Caitlin was right. As Dr. Peters told me years ago, I had to let Alex go. I also had to cut all of my girls some slack. I was holding them to the same standards I held myself, and it was destroying all of us. I was acting exactly like my mother.

In therapy, I learned to realize that my mother's expectations were completely unrealistic and had driven me to be a perfectionist. My mother was afraid of everything, so I was scared of nothing. My childhood and learned perfectionism drove me to try to be the best at everything. I wanted to feel exceptional. I was that overachieving middle child who tried to be the perfect kid so my parents might pay attention to me. My mother had issues from having an alcoholic father and losing her twin sister at an early age. She pushed my older sister and me to be successful. Good enough was never good enough. My sister rebelled, I was the model child, and my little brother was pampered. Rinse and repeat for a few decades, and the habit of striving for perfection was well ingrained to feel good—a vicious cycle.

I also remember being lonely as a child. I spent hours and hours reading under a huge shade tree in the backyard. I loved to read because it took me away from my reality. I dreamed about my perfect adult life. I would be a professional and have three perfect kids, a big house, nice cars, and an amazing husband. Somehow that didn't work out quite like my daydreams, but the girl in the tree believed in it.

Recovering from perfectionism is understanding the *why*. Why am I this way?

My mother regretted being too scared to leave our small town, so she pushed my sister and me to be the women she wanted to be and believed she would've been if only she took the opportunity to leave. I've heard the "if I had only taken the opportunity to be a secretary in Washington DC" story at least a thousand times. I believe her unrelenting pressure to be the best was grounded in her disappointments. I had to forgive her and then stop the cycle. Especially when talking with the girls, I had to think before I spoke. I had to hold them to a standard, but it didn't have to be perfect. I was driving them away, as my mother did me.

I also had to stop the negative self-talk by starting a mindfulness practice. I had to practice self-love. I *Recovering from perfectionism is understanding the why.* needed to remind myself daily about the things I've done well and forgive myself for the failures. I reminded myself that I have never failed. I've learned from my experiences and grown. I found myself becoming less judgmental, less arrogant, and kinder.

When Art first met me in 2012, he didn't like me. He thought I was an arrogant, self-righteous bitch. He was probably right. I was beating myself up so much about the chaos of my divorce that I had to keep reminding everyone around me how successful I was at everything else. The first time Art ran with my group of friends, I introduced myself as the vice chief of surgery at the local hospital, like it was a badge of success. He didn't care and thought I was full of myself.

I was my number one critic, and I was relentless. I had low self-esteem at the time because of my negative self-talk and perception of being a failure. Once I accepted that perfect was impossible and allowed myself not to strive for perfection every time, my world changed.

My perfectionism persisted because, on certain levels, it worked. It made me work harder in school and be a high achiever. It made me run harder and be more successful in my racing career. When I started my practice, it made me work longer hours because I had to be the best. Lori also suffered from perfectionism, so her habits fueled mine. We were a perfect collaborative workaholic pair. But when you're trying to be the perfect doctor, the perfect entrepreneur, the perfect wife, the perfect mother, and the perfect athlete, something has to give, and it did in spectacular fashion. That amount of stress slowly starts to kill you. Burnout is real. Superwoman Syndrome is impossible to keep up for decades, and only through reliving my childhood upbringing did I find the keys to recovery.

Superwoman Syndrome is impossible to keep up for decades, and only through reliving my childhood upbringing did I find the keys to recovery.

I learned to practice mindfulness and be present in the moment. I started using compassionate self-talk and challenging my negative self-judgments. These practices allowed me to accept that I couldn't be perfect at everything and I couldn't be everything for everybody.

Once I stopped beating myself up, I started to allow my girls to fail, then learn to get back up and grow. They would grow into the women they were meant to be. I stopped riding them to be the perfect kid I had in my fantasy world when I was a child. They didn't need to be perfect. They needed to be happy. For many years, I was unhappy because I was always striving for more. If I could reach this next level of affluence, popularity, wealth, I would be happy. It never happened. I always needed more. I was the proverbial glass that could never be filled. I learned to be happy with what I had.

Two things showed me that I was starting to recover from being a perfectionist.

First, in 2019, I took Alex to Cancun for a four-day weekend for her twenty-first birthday. Just the two of us. It was the most time that we'd spent together in almost seven years. We had a wonderful trip and talked about many things, but never once did I revisit the arguments of her teenage years and the pain we caused each other. The past was the past. I accepted that we might never be super close, but she was still my daughter, and I loved her. And I know on some level she loves me. We decided to be friends, and we'll take it from there. Dr. Peters was right—she was maturing and seeing me in a different light.

Second is that I'm writing this book. The perfectionist in me would never have allowed me to open this Pandora's box and certainly would never have put my story on display to the world for fear of rejection and judgment. I want my story of recovery from Superwoman Syndrome to inspire other women to be kinder to themselves and reevaluate their lives and goals. Balance is achievable if you take a long, hard look at your life, decide what's important, then use self-compassion and goal assessment to make a plan for you and your family.

13

RECOVERY IS POSSIBLE

Recovery from Superwoman Syndrome depends on first accepting that you are the core of your problem. Then you have to make a plan and do the work. Self-compassion and determination are the keys to a successful recovery. Ask for help and recruit a support team to help you. I have my family, friends, partners, clinical psychologist, and gynecologist on my team. Without them, my recovery wouldn't have been possible.

I found a lot of literature on both the physical and mental aspects of burnout, then set out on a quest to make a comprehensive plan.

I had to make drastic changes. First, I had to realize I couldn't do it all. It was okay to ask for help. I sat down with my family and the other doctors at work, and I let them know what was going on. I reduced my schedule to one that was much less ridiculous. I learned to be okay with decreasing my income for the sake of my health. I realized money didn't bring happiness or security, especially if it was ruining my health. We would survive and maybe even thrive. We didn't need more stuff; we needed more time.

I changed my diet. I asked for assistance with the household chores like laundry, dishes, cooking,

Ask for help and recruit a support team to help you.

and grocery shopping. I prayed more and started leaving things in God's hands instead of trying to fix everything. I started taking a multivitamin, B vitamins, an adrenal supplement, Vitamin D3, and progesterone. I practiced yoga and stopped doing HIIT classes. I started taking naps. I hydrated more and drank less alcohol. I started meditating and practiced mindfulness in every phase of my life. I got to the point where I wanted to run again. I found my husband attractive again. My sleep patterns normalized, and my irritability decreased. I started to feel like a human again!

It's okay to say you aren't okay and ask for help. Superwoman Syndrome is pathological, but you program yourself to believe that it's okay. How many times have you told yourself that you can do it all? It's time to reverse this trend! Stress can kill you, and Superwoman Syndrome makes everyone in the house miserable while you're trying to do it all.

So how do you break this cycle?

1. Talk to your doctor. Make sure nothing else is going on with your body. Reread the chapter on fatigue and the medical workup. Take notes.
2. Slow down your life. Learn to say no. Learn to ask for help, especially from your spouse and children. You didn't get married to wait on everyone. Marriage should be a partnership, and kids are not helpless. Remember that

you've trained your children to be worthless household help. You can retrain them to be helpful.

3. Delegate at work and decrease your schedule if at all possible. There are probably many things on your desk that someone else can do at least 75 percent as good a job as you, and that's okay! There are also things on your desk that can land in the circular file! Stop trying to do it all. Ditch the nine to five if you can—it allows you to focus on your life's purpose and your family.

4. Decrease or stop drinking alcohol. Read the chapter on overdrinking. It's incredible how many women use alcohol to medicate their anxiety and depression.

5. Change your diet. At the age of fifty, you cannot eat the same way you did as a teen. Half of your plate should be green or multi-colored with a mixture of raw and cooked vegetables. Any red meat should be lean and rare and not eaten more than once a week. Consult a nutritionist if you need help.

6. Add a multivitamin and adrenal supplement to your diet if your doctor approves. It's hard to get everything you need from your diet, and for me, the adrenal supplement was a life changer. It helped me recover more quickly.

7. Hydrate. Drink a minimum of sixty-four ounces of water, or at least half your body weight in ounces per day. Carry a water bottle with you everywhere.

8. Do low-impact exercise. Stretching, yoga, walking, slow running, swimming, and cycling with no time goals or extreme swings in heart rate can help you start feeling less fatigued.

9. Meditate, pray, journal. Find quiet time to focus on yourself. Breathing exercises are helpful too.

10. Don't sweat the small stuff. And most of it is small stuff. If it isn't going to matter five years from now, let it go.

11. It's okay to tell your kids, "No." They don't have to have a million activities that you have to drive them to, watch, and fund. Choose what they are genuinely passionate about and talk to them about how their activities affect the whole family.

12. Re-engage your sex life. Get closer to your spouse. Go on dates. Cuddle, flirt, and get to know each other in a biblical sense all over again. Kid-free vacations are allowed!

13. Get more organized. The chaos is stressful. Simplify. De-clutter. It's liberating to have organized cupboards. Use a centralized schedule for everyone and organize your family life.

14. Get your finances in order. Debt causes stress. Get rid of it, then save for a rainy day, the kids' college, and your retirement. Stop spending what you don't have. We all have so much stuff we don't need. We don't need more stuff; we need more time.

15. Unplug as much as you can. It probably sounds funny coming from a blogger, but start controlling your screen time. It is essential to set limits for TV, computer, email, and social media. That time is valuable and can be used to heal your mind, body, and soul.

16. Refocus on your plans in life. What do you feel your purpose is on this rock? Sit down and write out your goals for the next six months, one year, five years, ten years, and lifetime. Goal planning should include health, business, family, finances, and spiritual pursuits.

My last weeks in the office before I retired were bittersweet. I felt like George Bailey in the classic movie *It's a Wonderful Life*. I got cards, letters, phone calls, and visits from so many people who wanted to thank me for my help over the years.

One of my young female medical assistants wrote, "Dear Dr. Crane, I am so thankful for each and every moment I got to spend with you. You have taught me so many things, and most importantly, you have taught me to be more confident. You have loved us like your own family and not just employees. You inspire me every day, and I hope to be like you one day. Thank you for believing in me, even when I didn't believe in myself."

Another wrote, "I just wanted to say a massive thank you for all your help and guidance. It has been an honor to work and learn from you. Honestly, it is inspiring to see such a strong, confident, and quite frankly badass woman accomplish her dreams while being so humble and full of gratitude. You are an amazing role model, and I will miss chatting with you."

While I read their cards, I realized my work wasn't done. They still thought the Dr. Crane they saw each day in the office was the ideal role model. I never talked to them about how she fell apart piece by piece. Stephen Covey once said, "We judge ourselves by our intentions . . . while others judge us based on our behaviors." My intention was to retire and spend my time with my neglected family, to choose family over career. My intention was for my assistants and daughters to see this as an example of how your self-esteem didn't have to be wrapped up in your career.

I built that practice, and I felt like I left a lot of blood, sweat, and tears in the building; but when I looked at my finances and realized I could retire, my family goals won. I had to internalize the fact that my self-worth wasn't wrapped up in being Dr. Crane, and my life would be more balanced if I let the title and the associated chaos go. Lori was retiring as well. The office would go on without us. I wish them the best of luck and know they will be successful.

My practice blessed me immensely, and I felt very fulfilled and grateful. I left feeling content. I know that my medical career was at its pinnacle, and I said goodbye to Superwoman before she destroyed me mentally and physically. I look forward to the next stage of my life.

Girlfriend, it's okay to drop the S! Here I am a few years later, and I'm fit, fifty-plus, and fabulous. My life is so much healthier and balanced. I feel ten years younger. My marriage is fantastic, and my entire family is happier. Life is good!

You can get here too. Admitting to yourself that you can't do it all is the first step. Welcome to the rest of your life!

Once you've recovered, you'll wake up in the morning rested, happy, and thankful for all that you

Girlfriend, it's okay to drop the S!

have. Balance is attainable and marvelous. You'll go to work and have boundaries. You'll be fully present in the one task you decide to do at that moment.

I'm not perfect, and indeed, I feel like I have to work on myself every day, but I remind myself that it's okay to ask for help. Balance takes work. Money doesn't buy happiness. I don't have to win at everything. Communication is the key to all relationships. Aging well takes work, but sleep, a clean diet, hydration, and exercise are extremely important in keeping hormones balanced. It's okay to say no—it's the best word in the English language when used appropriately.

Recovery takes time and almost a complete rewiring of your brain. We were taught as little girls that mine was a generation of real feminine emancipation. Girls could do anything. But our mothers still waited on the family and gave us a gender role at home that was exactly like theirs. They programmed our inner critic and enforced that we needed to be everything for everybody.

How can we change these learned behaviors and start to find a balance between work, family, and community? Years ago, I heard that two women surgeons were job sharing, and I laughed at it at the time. Maybe that's an answer. Two moms and one job. Balance for some, insanity for others. Perhaps we change the expectations of men and their definition of the woman's role in the marriage, or better yet, make a marriage a true partnership where each spouse shares responsibilities, and there isn't a male or female role.

I believe we'll find answers with communication between recovered Superwomen and their adult children.

I sat down with my daughters and told them, "Don't follow my flawed example. You can be ambitious and successful and not sacrifice your health and sanity. You are three very different girls and need to find your own way by constantly asking, 'Why?' Why am I feeling guilty about taking time for myself? Why do I feel ashamed to ask for help when I'm overwhelmed? Why do I feel like I need to shoulder all the responsibility? Why does it have to be this way? How can I structure it better? Strive for balance in every part of your life. Raise your hand and ask for help. Realize that with age and family dynamics, life changes, and so the portions of each part change too. Life is full of seasons. Sometimes, it's a hard work season. Sometimes, it's an all-into-your-family season. Sometimes, it is even a self-love, it's-all-about-me season. Learn to adapt. Life is hard. You can't pour from an empty cup. Fill yours first, then get around to fill others. Choose to be happy! Choose to be the woman in *your* dreams—not mine or anyone else's!"

Let's rewire the next generation of women by showing them how to find balance, sanity, and overall health. Our daughters need patience, understanding of what season they're in, and help to stay healthy, balanced, and happy while achieving all of their dreams.

Let's change the job description of professional women and mothers. Only through valid societal changes can we all recover from Superwoman Syndrome and save the next generation of women from themselves.

RECOVERY RESOURCES

In this book, I mentioned significant lifestyle changes that enhanced my recovery from Superwoman Syndrome. Here are some additional resources that you may find helpful.

Before any diet, exercise program, or supplements are started, please seek the advice of your personal physician. Not all of the changes may be right for you, especially if you have some other underlying health conditions.

Adrenal supplements are helpful, especially in the early days of recovery. Here is a blog post with some more information on the specific supplements I utilized in my recovery: https://fitfiftyandfabulous.com/best-adrenal-fatigue-supplements/

Immune system supplements can be helpful to improve your overall health. Here are a few that can improve your gut health as well as improve your immune system: https://fitfiftyandfabulous.com/evaluating-immune-boosting-supplements/

The Metabolism Plan by Lyn-Genet Recitas contains a vegan cleanse and anti-inflammatory diet that I personally follow. More information at https://lyngenet.com/the-metabolism-plan/

Stress Relief Meditation discusses the basics of meditation and how to incorporate it into your life. Available on Amazon at https://amzn.to/3tRUbYy

How to Stop Overdrinking is a short guide on how to plan your drinking, as discussed in Chapter five. Available on Amazon at https://amzn.to/37dTIqa

If you find that you are unable to plan your drinking, quit drinking. You don't have to suffer alone. There are lots of programs to help you, like Alcoholics Anonymous at https://www.aa.org/.

Are you depressed? A great first resource is this quiz that you can discuss with your doctor or therapist: https://psychcentral.com/quizzes/depression-quiz/.

The Money Cleanse was written for my daughters. It will help you change your attitude towards money, get out of debt, and encourage you to accumulate savings. Available on Amazon at https://amzn.to/3aoRjLj.

A gratitude journal is a powerful way to reset your mindset each day. The one I use is *Good Days Start with Gratitude*. Available on Amazon at https://amzn.to/3aYozI0.

The Art of Self-Love is a guide to reprogramming your inner critic and loving yourself unconditionally. Available on Amazon at https://amzn.to/2LQzTh3.

Beginner Power Yoga Poses can help you start a restorative exercise regimen. Available on Amazon at https://amzn.to/37e8Nrr.

My blog, FitFiftyandFabulous.com, is updated often and contains helpful resources that may be helpful in guiding your recovery.

Please reach out with any questions or ideas for additional resources that I can share with my tribe. It takes a village! Marybeth@FitFiftyandFabulous.com

Updates to this book and frequently asked questions will be available at DroptheS.com

ACKNOWLEDGMENTS

"Gratitude makes sense of our past, brings peace for today, and creates a vision for tomorrow."

—Melody Beattie

This book was the culmination of a long recovery process that could not have occurred without the loving support of my family, friends, and the North Texas medical community. The story unwound over a period of more than ten years, and I'm so thankful for the people who stuck with me and encouraged me along my turbulent journey. Writing this book was the best therapy I could have had.

Thank you to my parents for instilling in me the New England values of hard work, grit, and perseverance. Our family dynamics were often tumultuous, but your love was always unconditional. My father has passed away, and I miss him every day, but I remember one of his last statements before he went to our Lord was, "It was worth it." I think he meant that any of the struggles of his life were worth the legacy he left behind in my sister, Terry, me, and my little brother, Rob. He was proud of all of us.

I especially thank my dear, sweet husband, Art Atchison, for being with me through every step of my crash and burn, then my recuperation. Your support was essential for recovery. Art, you never gave up on me and kept reinforcing how much you loved me even when I was a hot mess. Thank you for your patience and love. I love you more each day.

I want to thank my three daughters, Alexandra, Caitlin, and Sasha, for inspiring me to be a better mother and example for them. You motivate me to seek balance so that the cycle of Superwoman Syndrome doesn't continue with the next generation. I love each of you so much.

I thank my mentor, Dr. Bruce Werber. Without your encouragement and assistance, I don't think I would have taken the leap of faith to pursue podiatry. You changed my life's trajectory and only for the better. Now as my close friend, you are often my sounding board and chief confidant. I love that you are still in my life.

I would be extremely remiss if I didn't thank Rem Jackson, the founder of Top Practices. Rem, you've been with me as a coach and friend through this entire saga. Lori introduced us, and we were part of your first mastermind meeting. You encouraged me to write this book after talking me off the ledge so many times. Your support and profound insight have been an integral part of my success and my recovery. At the Top Practices Summit in 2019, you gave me your stage to tell my story, and that led directly to this book.

Rem introduced me to Nancy Erickson, The Book Professor®, who coached me through writing, editing, and finally publishing this book. Nancy, thank you for never giving up on my story. Without you, this book would still be in my journaling notebook. I love that you believe everyone has a book in them, and you helped me make mine a reality. If anyone else is interested in book coaching, check out www.bookprofessor. com. Nancy was wonderful to work with, and she let my voice shine in my writing.

I especially need to thank my dear friend since junior high, Colleen Schiermeyer, who stuck with me on this rollercoaster ride. You were front and center for this implosion and subsequent recovery. Colleen, growing up together in Rhode Island and then moving to Texas with me, you understood the dynamics of our joint history and were always available to listen any time I needed to rant. Two RI girls in Texas who stuck together. I'll always be grateful for your listening ear and your shoulder to cry on.

In closing, there are no words to adequately thank Lori Cerami. Our stories are interwoven. I never would've achieved the level of success in business without you. Your friendship has been incredibly valuable to me through the good times and the bad. Our brains put together are collaborative and powerful. One day, I hope you'll put your story on paper as well. I continue to miss Elise every day, as I know you do as well. She will never be forgotten. The Swim4Elise foundation is her legacy.

There are so many other people to thank that I can't possibly include them all. All the past and present members of the Top Practices Top Performers Mastermind group: Thank you for helping me troubleshoot so many ideas and for accompanying me on my journey. All the members of Lake Grapevine Runners and Walkers who supported my running problem and my practice for over twenty-five years: running truly is group therapy. All the past and present doctors and staff at Foot and Ankle Associates of North Texas: Your hard work and dedication allowed me to shine. Your empathy permitted me to step back and change gears in my last year of private practice. Thank you for that levity. The Gateway Church single mother's ministry: You facilitated the path to find my way back to the Lord and encouraged me as I healed from my divorce. I felt your love and acceptance along the way. Forgiveness of myself and my ex allowed me to fall in love again.

None of this would've been possible without all of these people, and I am extremely grateful to each and every one who contributed to this journey. I hope my story helps others along the way on similar expeditions.

I am humbled, blessed, and grateful. Thank you all.

ABOUT THE AUTHOR

Dr. Crane is a retired board-certified podiatric foot and ankle surgeon. She specialized in sports medicine in private practice for over twenty-five years and successfully built a multi-million-dollar private practice from humble beginnings.

She is passionate about holistic wellness, which can help your physical, mental, spiritual, and financial health. She authors a blog on women's health and wellness issues as well as relationships, communication, and the issues surrounding the lovely aging process at www.fitfiftyandfabulous.com.

Dr. Crane has been a competitive distance runner for more than forty years. She's completed more than twenty marathons, a dozen or so Half Ironmans, and two full Ironman Triathlons. She is blessed with three wonderful daughters and two stepdaughters, and a loyal male dog. Her husband is truly a saint.

Contact her at marybeth@fitfiftyandfabulous.com. Follow her @myrundoc on Twitter, @fitfiftyandfabulous on Facebook, and @myrundoc.crane on Instagram.

CPSIA information can be obtained
at www.ICGtesting.com
Printed in the USA
JSHW051706030721
16554JS00001B/7